A Touch of Diabetes

Third Edition

A Straightforward Guide for People Who Have Type 2 Diabetes

Lois Jovanovic-Peterson, M.D.,

Charles M. Peterson, M.D.,

and Morton B. Stone

JOHN WILEY & SONS, INC.

New York · Chichester · Weinheim · Brisbane · Singapore · Toronto

The information contained in this book is not intended to serve as a replacement for professional medical advice. Any use of the information in this book is at the reader's discretion. The author and the publisher specifically disclaim any and all liability arising directly or indirectly from the use or application of any information contained in this book. A health care professional should be consulted regarding your specific situation.

ISBN 0-471-34754-X

Printed in the United States of America

10 9 8 7 6 5 4 3

About the Authors

LOIS JOVANOVIC-PETERSON, M.D., is director and chief scientific officer of the Sansum Medical Research Institute. A board-certified internist and endocrinologist, she has served as the chair of the Council on Pregnancy of the American Diabetes Association. In 1995, she was the recipient of the American Diabetes Association's Outstanding Physician Clinician Award, and in 1998 she received the Zitter Award for Diabetes Disease Management Leadership. Her research has been in the field of diabetes and pregnancy, and islet transplantation.

Dr. Jovanovic-Peterson has written hundreds of articles on diabetes and authored or co-authored 24 books on diabetes, including *The Diabetic Woman, Diabetes Self-Care Method,* and *Hormones: The Woman's Answerbook.*

CHARLES M. PETERSON, M.D., is program director, Blood Diseases Program in the Division of Blood Diseases and Blood Resources of the National Heart Lung Blood Institute of the National Institutes of Health. He pioneered the use of home blood glucose monitoring and the use of the hemoglobin A1c test as a monitor of blood glucose control. These efforts along with improved use of insulin and other therapies were critical in making possible the numerous studies that now prove the importance of maintaining near normal blood glucose levels to avoid the complications of diabetes.

Dr. Peterson has authored or co-authored more than 350 scientific publications and over 20 books on diabetes, including the first two editions of this book, *Take Charge of Your Diabetes* (published by Morton B. Stone), and *The Diabetes Self-Care Method.* Dr. Peterson resides in Potomac, Maryland, with his wife Karen and children Caroline and Alexander.

MORTON B. STONE co-authored the first two editions of this book and was a co-author with Dr. Lois Jovanovic-Peterson of *Managing Your Gestational Diabetes.* In 1997, he was diagnosed with Type 2 diabetes. Stone formerly was the founder and editorial director of the magazine *Diabetes in the News* and has written many educational booklets for people with diabetes. He was one of the founders and is an honorary member of the American Association of Diabetes Educators.

Contents

	Editor's Note	9
CHAPTER 1	You Have a Touch of Diabetes	11
CHAPTER 2	Diabetes: Past, Present, and Future	19
CHAPTER 3	What Diabetes Is and What It Isn't	23
CHAPTER 4	Your Body and Blood Glucose	29
CHAPTER 5	Your Emotions and Diabetes	35
CHAPTER 6	Food: It's Your Choice	43
CHAPTER 7	Exercise: The Options are Plentiful	63
CHAPTER 8	Medications	75
CHAPTER 9	Monitoring Your Health	93
CHAPTER 10	Sex and Sexuality	109
CHAPTER 11	Complications	121
CHAPTER 12	Dear Diary	131
CHAPTER 13	To Learn More About It	135
	Glossary of Diabetes Terms	145
	Bibliography	155
	Index	159

Editor's Note

Morton B. Stone, one of the authors of *A Touch of Diabetes,* was diagnosed in 1997 as having Type 2 diabetes. His experiences as a person with a "touch" of diabetes (newly diagnosed) may well mirror your own responses to diagnosis and the demands for a change in lifestyle in order to control this disease.

Stone has maintained a journal that reflects his responses not only to the recommendations of his health care professionals but also to the advice offered in this book. We have taken excerpts from this journal and included them in this 3rd edition of *A Touch of Diabetes.* No doubt you will be able to identify with his reactions and comments, since they are probably very similar to your own.

CHAPTER I

You Have a Touch of Diabetes

WHEN YOUR DOCTOR FIRST TOLD YOU that you had diabetes, how did you react?

"I don't believe it. I don't have any symptoms."

"No, there must be a mistake. I feel fine."

"Why me? I've been in perfect health."

Or did you say, "It can't be bad.... Isn't it just a touch of diabetes?"

Your doctor probably said your blood glucose levels were just a bit above normal. Perhaps your weight, too, was above normal. Was it described as a "touch" of diabetes?

Your doctor may have said your body's metabolism had misfired, resulting in a rise in your blood glucose levels (also known as blood sugar levels). Because of this, your doctor suggested a few changes in your lifestyle: you need to watch what and how much you eat, get more exercise, and lose any extra weight you've been carrying around the last few years.

Whether this advice came recently or you heard it years ago when you were first diagnosed with Type 2 diabetes, it is good advice to follow. However, knowing something is good for you—and doing it—are two different things. We know it is challenging to alter eating habits, to change a sedentary lifestyle, to get rid of extra pounds. But it is worth it.

Recent research has shown the necessity of making the diagnosis of diabetes earlier in the disease process. If we wait too long, high blood glucose levels cause complications. Thus, the American Diabetes Association has lowered the diagnosis threshold to make sure that treatment is offered *before* it is too late to prevent complications. The new diagnosis criterion is a fasting plasma glucose level equal to or more than 126 mg/dl (7.0 mmol/L) on two or more tests.

Unfortunately, too many people do little to control their diabetes unless they develop one of the complications of diabetes. Sadly, these people have missed a wonderful opportunity, because it is what you do today and in the days, months, and years to come, that has the most effect on preventing or postponing complications. The complications of diabetes are indeed a strong motivation for people to take action to control their disease. We'll talk more about the risks of diabetes throughout this book, particularly in Chapter 11. For now, though, please know that Type 2 diabetes is serious, but there are proven ways to minimize its impact, which you'll learn here.

As we've mentioned, some people who are told they have a touch of diabetes are not motivated to change their life and control it. They come up with lots of reasons to postpone action. They believe scientists will develop a miracle drug to cure diabetes one of these days. Unfortunately, such a miracle drug does not exist and it's unlikely that one will be developed to cure Type 2 diabetes.

They believe their diabetes will just go away if they deny it and ignore it. Sadly, this assumption, too, is wrong! Diabetes is permanent. It will be with you the rest of your life.

They believe it is the doctor's responsibility to control their diabetes by designing a program to reduce blood glucose levels. Although doctors can design excellent diabetes management plans for you, it is up to you to implement the plan. This requires a bit of discipline, but in the long run, it is well worth the effort. With diabetes, you, rather than your health care professional, have the major role in determining the success of your management plan.

They believe that it is too late and they are too old to make changes in their lives. It is never too late to take control of diabetes—even if you have already developed some complications. Blood glucose control can provide immediate benefits, today and in the future, even if you never return to "perfect" blood sugar levels.

Your doctor will establish a "normal" range of blood sugar levels for you. And you can start an exercise and weight-control program no matter what your age or challenges. Each of the parts of the diabetes management program can be tailored to your needs, tastes, and physical status.

Of course, medical advice and a diabetes management plan isn't beneficial until it is followed. Again, you must decide to implement these recommendations. You're in charge of your diabetes, but you can get lots of help. Your diabetes health care team, family members, friends, and other people with diabetes are all excellent supporters. But, it's up to you to heed the advice and make the changes in your lifestyle that will help keep your blood glucose levels within the normal range.

You will have to make changes in your lifestyle. But you'll also have many options regarding those changes. For example, there are choices to make about the foods you eat and choices involving the exercise you do. With these choices and changes, you'll be able to take control, not only of your diabetes, but also your life. And by sticking with a plan, you'll lower your blood glucose levels and reduce the risks of developing complications.

You may feel overwhelmed at first, but please remember:

1. Despite this book's title and what your doctor may have told you, there really is no such thing as "A Touch of Diabetes." You have been diagnosed as having Type 2 diabetes. Diabetes is a metabolic disorder that cannot be ignored, even if a person's blood glucose levels are only slightly elevated at the time of diagnosis.

2. You have the major responsibility for controlling your diabetes and your blood glucose levels. No one else can do the things needed to manage your diabetes.

3. As we've mentioned, there are a variety of choices available concerning your food and physical activities. For example, a sugary

food is not out of the question if your blood glucose is in good control and it is part of a well balanced meal. (In Chapter 6, you'll learn how to count the carbohydrates in that food as part of your daily allowance.) And, you can mow the lawn, do housework, or walk to the store as part of your exercise program, instead of going to the health club.

Your new lifestyle should be one that everyone in your family can enjoy. Your meals can be appetizing as well as healthful. Typical eating plans are appealing to adults and children. Exercise plans, too, can be shared by all ages.

4. You have lots of resources. You have your professional diabetes health care team members: your physician, nurse educator, dietitian, a counselor, pharmacist, and an exercise expert (sometimes referred to as a "personal trainer"). Depending on where you live, these people may not always be available in person, but you can learn lots from a phone call.

There are also national and local branches of the diabetes association, hospital diabetes centers, community centers, and local service organizations. And don't forget your family and friends, who should be encouraged to learn about and support your new lifestyle.

5. There are changes to be made in your life, but they don't have to be difficult. A diabetes management plan emphasizes a healthy and exciting lifestyle, one where you're in charge. Genes and lifestyle have a lot to do with developing Type 2 diabetes. You can't do anything about those genes, but you can change your lifestyle.

Keep in mind that changes are just that—changes. They are not static, and you'll be making them continuously as you get older and your body changes. What works today may not be effective tomorrow, so be prepared to grow in your understanding of your health and change accordingly. But that's something everyone needs to do, diabetes or not. You'll just have more awareness and control than others.

From Morton's Journal

Why me??? Of all the people in the world, how could this happen to me?

I have been writing about diabetes and diabetes management for the past three decades and I had been giving readers of my writings advice on how they should take care of themselves and even prevent the occurrence of diabetes. Could it be guilt by association? Could I have picked up the symptoms of diabetes by being exposed to all of the facts, recommendations, and advice on diabetes self management?

I didn't believe it when my doctor said that I had Type 2 diabetes. "Not true," I said. "Maybe my blood glucose was a little bit high...but that must be due to the fact that I had put on a few pounds in the last couple of months since I retired. Or it could have been due to the stress that I was placed under not only when I retired but also when I moved from familiar surroundings in Chicago to the sunny climate of Sarasota, Florida."

My verbal response to my doctor's pronouncement was to say, "The tests must be wrong." The doctor assured me that they were not, and advised me to come back in three months for another blood glucose measurement, plus a hemoglobin A1c test [more about this test in Chapter 9].

When I returned home, I had a little talk with myself and said that maybe I should listen to my own advice...you know, all of the stories on how to self-manage diabetes through diet and exercise.

As most people find out, it's one thing to say diet and exercise and another thing to do these activities on a routine basis.

So (even though I did not admit that I might have Type 2 diabetes) I started to think more about diet and exercise. The weather in Sarasota is far more conducive to exercise than it was in my former home in Chicago (particularly during the winter...and sometimes fall and spring). So out came the bicycle and the swimming trunks and lawn mower. Unfortunately, when the local temperature moved into the 90s, the effort required to mow and bicycle even fairly modest distances became "heroic." The swimming pool was the exercise choice with first priority, and soon became a daily habit.

Dieting was another matter entirely. As I re-read the articles I wrote on food choices, I reminded myself to cut down on eating extra fatty foods, and to eat more chicken and fish than beef, lamb, and pork. It was even easier to cut out sweet, high-fat desserts (which I really didn't care for anyway).

I didn't do a thing about portion control, nor was I about to count calories, carbohydrates, points, or exchanges.

And I didn't bother to check the bathroom scales to see how well, or how poorly I was doing.

Those first three months flew by, and the next thing I knew I was back in my doctor's office for a checkup (after having blood drawn for analysis the week before).

The news was less than pleasant. My blood glucose (fasting) had risen rather than dropped. My weight dropped all of two pounds. The only good news, I stated, was that my hemoglobin A1c was below 7 (by a fraction). It must be "glucose intolerance" (the new, accepted name for borderline diabetes), I said proudly.

You have Type 2 diabetes, my doctor said. No way, I said. It's just a little intolerance. Again the doctor prescribed diet and exercise and recommended another evaluation in three months.

I left the doctor's office secure with my self-diagnosis. "What's a little glucose intolerance?" I thought. After all, my hemoglobin A1c was still in the okay range.

I proceeded to follow the plan of action I had installed prior to this doctor's visit and pretty well maintained it during the next three months. Going out to dine at restaurants was a real challenge (since I did not even admit to myself that I had diabetes), but I tried to make reasonably healthy food choices. Having a martini or two before dinner, however, was a habit that was hard to break or even modify. I kept telling myself that many recent medical reports said that having a drink or two each day was a healthy habit.

Those three months passed quickly and once again I was at the doctor's office (following a visit to the lab for a blood test). "Well," my doctor said, "your fasting blood glucose has moved up again—to 170 mg/dl (9.4 mmol/L)—and your hemoglobin A1c is now above 7." I didn't hear how much above 7 the level was, but the fact that it was above 7 was the clincher for me.

"Oh boy, I do have Type 2 diabetes," I exclaimed...like I had never heard my doctor say anything during the two previous office visits. It was like someone had turned on the lights in a dark room. The facts cut through all my layers of "informed" denial, and I accepted that of all things, I had diabetes.

After a few moments I asked the doctor what his recommended plan of attack....err...management was.

He checked my chart (weight, blood pressure, etc.) and said that I certainly knew enough about diabetes management to apply the principles to my own life. However, he pointed out that my own "flexible" approach to diet and exercise was not too effective in either lowering my weight or my blood glucose levels.

He said that I might want to pay more attention to the recommendations in this book (to which I replied that I would have to re-read it) and perhaps may benefit from the addition of a low dose of oral hypoglycemic medication to more closely control my blood glucose. He suggested that I might want to purchase a blood glucose meter and use it to monitor just how well (or poorly) my efforts were doing.

As I left the doctor's office, I muttered to myself, I do have more than a "Touch of Diabetes."

CHAPTER 2

Diabetes:
Past, Present, and Future

THE MEDICAL NAME for this disease is *diabetes mellitus.* The term *diabetes* comes from the Greek word that means to siphon or to flow through. The term *mellitus* comes from the Latin word that means honey or sweet.

Diabetes appears to have been around a long time. Ancient Egyptians reported the disease and even developed some crude treatments for it. Diabetes was also noted in Roman writings and in ancient India, where vigorous exercise was recommended as treatment. (Interestingly, exercise remains the cornerstone of treatment programs today.)

In the Middle Ages, medical experts called Pisse Prophets used their sense of smell or taste to diagnose this sugar disease from patients' urine. Sadly, there was little hope for the person who had diabetes. People with Type 1 diabetes (the insulin-dependent variety) continued to lose weight and energy, and usually died shortly after diagnosis. People with Type 2 diabetes would usually develop one or more of the major diabetes complications, amputation of limbs, blindness, and even death from heart and circulatory disease.

The tragedies continued to the early part of this century. It was not until Drs. Banting and Best discovered how to extract insulin from animals (cows and pigs) and use the insulin to treat diabetes that things changed. The first people to really benefit from this breakthrough received treatment only 75 to 80 years ago.

In the 1940s and '50s, many medical professionals recommended that blood glucose levels should be maintained at an above-normal level. This allowed patients to feel good and lowered their risks for low blood sugar attacks (low blood sugar is also known as hypoglycemia), but it also did little to prevent complications, we later learned. Oral hypoglycemic agents were first introduced in the 1960s, and the insulin-infusion pump (used by people with Type 1 diabetes to inject insulin instead of needles and syringes) was perfected only in the late 1980s.

By the 1970s, many physicians started to believe that people with diabetes needed to keep their blood sugar levels in the normal range. This, at least in theory at the time, reduced the risks for developing major complications.

The first convenient urine sugar test was produced at the end of World War II, but it wasn't until 1980 that people with diabetes were able to monitor blood glucose levels at home. In fact, the tools for keeping blood glucose in the normal range and in "tight" control were not available until after 1980. That's when self blood glucose monitoring, human insulin, multiple insulin injection plans, and second-generation oral agents all became available.

Then, in 1993, a nationwide scientific study called the Diabetes Control and Complications Trial proved the value of keeping tight blood glucose to prevent, delay, or lessen the severity of the major complications of diabetes.

In Search of the Best Eating Plan

For many years, the diabetes eating plan was controversial among doctors. Before the 1940s, your diet would have varied from a starvation plan, to an all-vegetable plan, to a high-fat plan. Carbohydrates in particular were not acceptable until recently, when people with Type 2 diabetes were told to eat large amounts of complex carbohydrates and fiber, but to limit fat.

Today, if blood glucose is in good control, the person with diabetes can enjoy a wide variety of food, including an occasional sweet treat when it is part of a well-balanced meal. Fats are limited for most, but there still is no clear consensus about how much total carbohydrate is appropriate. The main thing is that your diet works for you and keeps your blood sugar, blood lipids or fats, and blood pressure in the target range agreed upon by you and your doctor.

New Evidence about Exercise

Exercise recommendations have also been the subject of a number of recent changes in diabetes management. Experts used to tell people with diabetes to do 30 to 40 minutes of moderate exercise, three or four times a week. Some people were told to exercise every day. Recommended activities included walking, biking, swimming, or even competitive games, such as tennis. The goal was to burn calories, lower blood glucose, and improve physical fitness.

In 1994, however, new evidence suggested changes were appropriate about exercise recommendations. Studies showed that exercise did not have to be limited to a 30- or 40-minute session of walking or working out at a health club, for instance. Equal benefits can be gained through mild to moderate physical activity, such as walking, housework, and mowing the lawn, for short periods (10 minutes) three to four times daily, every day of the week.

Further studies reveal that moderately intense workouts, 30 to 40 minutes each and three to four times a week, seem to increase the life spans of those who exercise compared with those who do only mild to moderate physical activity.

You, your doctor, and a nutrition expert should discuss your personalized eating and exercise plans to determine what is right for you. This book, too, will offer suggestions. As you embark on an exercise program, perhaps for the first time ever, remember that everyone is different. What's appropriate for your neighbor may not be right for you. So start slowly and enjoy the many benefits of exercise.

CHAPTER 3

What Diabetes Is and What It Isn't

AS MENTIONED EARLIER, diabetes mellitus is a disease in which there are above normal levels of glucose (sugar) in the bloodstream. This glucose sometimes spills over from the kidneys into the urine.

There are two major kinds of diabetes mellitus: Type 1 and Type 2. Each is different and requires a different management program. In the past, Type 1 diabetes was called insulin-dependent diabetes mellitus (IDDM) or juvenile-onset diabetes, and Type 2 was called noninsulin-dependent diabetes mellitus (NIDDM) or adult-onset diabetes. However, these terms are misleading. An estimated 40 percent of people with Type 2 diabetes use insulin. Moreover, children are being diagnosed with Type 2 diabetes. Another form of diabetes is gestational diabetes, which occurs in some women during pregnancy. Finally, some people have a condition called impaired glucose tolerance, which is sometimes referred to as borderline diabetes.

Between 10 and 15 percent of the people with diabetes have Type 1 diabetes. Eighty-five percent or more have Type 2 diabetes, and half of these don't know they have it. Approximately 2 to 12 percent of pregnant women develop gestational diabetes.

About Type 1 Diabetes
Although you may have Type 2 diabetes and don't require insulin, it is helpful to learn a bit about Type 1 diabetes. Type 1 diabetes usually develops during childhood or adolescence, although

adults do develop this form of diabetes. It develops over a period of years and often goes undiagnosed until severe symptoms occur, usually in the form of rapid and dramatic weight loss.

In Type 1 diabetes, the insulin-producing cells in the pancreas gland no longer secrete insulin. When these cells stop working, supplemental insulin becomes necessary to sustain life. A malfunction in the immune system seems to destroy these insulin-producing cells. It is believed to start with several genetic defects that may be triggered into action by a viral infection. To fight the virus, the immune system kills the viral invaders. But the immune system fails to shut off once the virus has been conquered. Instead, it goes on to attack and destroy healthy cells in the body, including the insulin-producing cells of the pancreas. Eventually, all of these cells are destroyed, which stops the body's ability to produce insulin.

The management plan for Type 1 diabetes usually includes multiple daily injections of insulin (two or more a day), by syringe or insulin pump. People with Type 1 diabetes must adhere strictly to their eating and exercise schedules to match the action and duration of action of the supplemental insulin. They must also monitor their blood glucose levels frequently, usually four to eight times a day. Oral hypoglycemic agents are not effective in Type 1 diabetes.

With Type 1 diabetes, not only is there increased risk for low blood glucose attacks, but there is risk of very high elevated blood glucose levels (called *hyperglycemia*), which can trigger complications such as ketosis and ketoacidosis. These complications can result in coma and unconsciousness in extreme cases. There are also long-term concerns about the major complications of diabetes affecting vision, nerves, the circulatory system, and kidney function.

About Type 2 Diabetes

The vast majority of people with diabetes have Type 2 diabetes. In this type of diabetes, your body does not produce enough insulin or it may be resistant to the insulin that it does produce. Without enough usable insulin, glucose in the bloodstream accumulates and can eventually damage nerves and blood vessels throughout the body.

There is strong evidence that Type 2 diabetes is an inherited disease. If you have Type 2 diabetes, there is a great likelihood that your parent, grandparent, or an aunt or uncle also has or had the disease.

Type 2 diabetes usually—but not always—develops in adults over the age of 40. Women who have given birth to babies weighing more than 9 pounds are also susceptible to developing Type 2 diabetes. Body weight also seems to be a factor. About 85 percent of newly diagnosed cases occur in people who are overweight or clinically obese at the time of diagnosis.

In most cases, Type 2 diabetes develops silently, with no easily recognizable symptoms during the development stage of this disease. Perhaps that was your experience. Often, it is diagnosed only when people undergoing physical examinations have their fasting blood glucose measured. In others, the diagnosis is easily confirmed when symptoms do appear and damage to the body's organs has already begun.

Management plans for Type 2 diabetes vary according to how severe its effects are and how committed you are to making healthy choices and staying with them. At first, Type 2 diabetes can be managed by regulating diet and exercise, in addition to blood glucose monitoring. One of your first goals will be to lose any extra weight and keep it off through regular exercise. You'll also monitor your blood glucose regularly to adjust your food and exercise, all to help keep your blood glucose within a normal range as defined by your doctor.

If blood glucose levels do not normalize, the doctor will usually prescribe an oral hypoglycemic agent to help. This drug will not work on its own. It needs to be combined with an eating and exercise plan.

For some people with Type 2 diabetes, insulin injections, either alone or in combination with an oral agent, may be needed to keep blood glucose levels within the normal range. Type 2 patients who take insulin are referred to as "insulin-requiring" patients rather than "insulin-dependent," the term often still used in Type 1 diabetes.

If you do not need insulin or an oral agent to help keep your blood glucose levels in the normal range, you are probably not at high risk for low blood glucose attacks, ketosis, or acidosis.

The complications associated with Type 2 diabetes are somewhat linked to the complications associated with obesity: heart attacks, cardiovascular problems, and hypertension. That's why weight loss is such an important goal for many people with Type 2 diabetes. Other long-term complications that can occur if blood glucose is not properly controlled include impotence, retinopathy, and neuropathy. We'll discuss more about these later in the book.

About Gestational Diabetes

Gestational diabetes may develop in previously healthy women during pregnancy. It can be detected with a blood glucose test done in about the 24th week of pregnancy. As mentioned earlier, gestational diabetes occurs in 2 to 12 percent of pregnant women. Although gestational diabetes requires intensive treatment during the pregnancy, it usually disappears when the baby is born. Treatment is usually dietary management but may include insulin injections and frequent blood glucose measurements.

Women who develop gestational diabetes are at increased risk for developing Type 2 diabetes later in life. This means women who have had gestational diabetes should have their fasting plasma glucose measured during regular physical checkups. Because weight is often a factor in Type 2 diabetes, at-risk women should make a special effort to lose extra weight if they had been overweight before or during pregnancy.

What Diabetes is Not

Diabetes is not a disease you catch from or give to your spouse, friends, or coworkers. You may have inherited a genetic tendency for developing the disease, which may also be passed to your children.

Diabetes is not a disease you get from eating too much sugar.

Sugar by itself does not cause diabetes, but it may send blood glucose levels higher than normal, just as other foods can. Table sugar just gets into the bloodstream faster than complex carbohydrates, protein, or fats.

Diabetes is not a disease that can be cured with a miracle drug. Although scientists are working hard to find a cure for diabetes, they have not been successful. They have had some success in experimental methods that may prevent or delay Type 1 diabetes. For some people with Type 2 diabetes, the closest thing to a cure is to lose excess weight and keep it off. A 10-pound weight loss can significantly lower blood glucose levels. Normalizing weight can sometimes completely eliminate the symptoms of the disease.

Diabetes is not a disease that will go away. Unlike pneumonia, the common cold, and other conditions that can be eliminated by treatment, medication, or time, diabetes is permanent. You will have it for the rest of your life. However, by making good choices that help to bring your blood glucose levels into the normal range, you can plan to enjoy a long, healthy, productive life. Plus, you may have an advantage. Understanding the importance of managing your weight and following a sensible eating plan and exercise regimen goes a long way in helping you live longer than people who are not so enlightened.

From Morton's Journal

The more you know about diabetes the better able you will be to handle the management of this disease. I've been fortunate to have worked in this field for the past three decades and I have read almost everything that has been published about diabetes. I still read as much as I can, and I attend lectures and talks about diabetes developments. What is exciting is the fact that medical science is discovering new things about diabetes and diabetes management at an ever-increasing pace. What was current two years ago may be obsolete today.

CHAPTER 4

Your Body and Blood Glucose

DIABETES DEVELOPS WHEN our body does not have, or cannot use, the hormone called insulin to help glucose get into cells to make energy. Sometimes no insulin is produced by the specific cells in the pancreas, as in Type 1 diabetes. Sometimes there isn't enough insulin to meet the body's needs. More often, though, the insulin produced doesn't work properly because of a condition known as insulin resistance.

Once inside the cells, glucose serves as fuel to keep the body working efficiently. Without enough glucose, cells just don't work properly. Without any glucose for fuel, cells die.

Insulin comes from beta cells in the pancreas gland or from injections of manufactured insulin. Glucose comes from the food we eat. The body digests most of the food we eat and converts it into glucose, the simplest form of sugar. The glucose then enters the bloodstream and circulates until needed as fuel by the cells.

Under normal conditions, the required quantities of glucose are matched with required amounts of insulin. These partners then move to and are absorbed into cells where the glucose is burned as fuel, providing your body with needed energy.

If there is a foul-up in the system, two conditions result: First, unused glucose stays in the blood and continues to pile up; and second, unused glucose is converted into fat cells, which serve as storehouses or reserves that can be used during periods of starvation. (In early history, this natural storage system worked well in the face of regular periods of starvation. But today, most people are not starving so fat layers build, year after overfed year, and obesity and weight problems are common.)

In addition to vitamins, minerals, and fiber, food is composed of three major components: carbohydrates (simple and complex), proteins, and fats (saturated, monounsaturated, and polyunsaturated).

The body converts carbohydrates, proteins, and fats into glucose. This conversion occurs at different speeds, depending on the nutrient. Simple carbohydrates, like sucrose or table sugar, are the fastest to enter the bloodstream as glucose. Complex carbohydrates take a bit more time. Fats and proteins are digested more slowly before they are converted to glucose.

Blood glucose levels change according to the amount of glucose in the bloodstream at any particular time. For example, if you eat a lot of simple carbohydrates, the glucose will enter your bloodstream very quickly, sending blood glucose levels soaring.

If you eat lots of food of any kind, your blood glucose levels, over time, will rise above normal. Conversely, if you cut down on the amount of food you eat, your blood glucose will reflect this by staying lower.

These levels also change as glucose leaves the bloodstream to enter the cells as fuel. The more active you are, the more fuel the cells need so more glucose leaves the bloodstream. If your body is burning a great amount of fuel, such as when you exercise strenuously, a number of things can happen:

1. If you haven't eaten much, there's a particular risk that your body will use up the glucose in your bloodstream. As a result, blood glucose levels will drop, sometimes quite rapidly and to quite low levels. That's when hypoglycemia occurs, something to avoid. It is also why it is important that your doctor adjust your oral medications or insulin injections when you start an exercise program.

2. If the energy demands are not intense and continue over time, exercise will force your body to turn to its reserves (fat cells) and use them for fuel. That's very beneficial for those of us who need to lose weight.

As we've said, many people with Type 2 diabetes carry some extra weight in the form of stored fat. If that's your situation, make the fat stores work for you by exercising moderately on a regular schedule and restricting the number of calories in your eating plan.

Blood glucose levels may also go up or down if you take insulin injections or an oral hypoglycemic agent, especially if you don't coordinate your eating and exercise schedule with your medication schedule. For instance, if you skip a meal but take your medication, either orally or by injection, at the regular time, you are apt to send your blood glucose levels down into the danger zone. If you over-exercise, or if you skip your regular exercise, your blood glucose levels will reflect that change in your activities.

Stress or even a common cold can affect blood glucose levels. So if you are experiencing a lot of stress or have a minor illness, your blood glucose levels may go very high—unless, of course, you make adjustments in your management program. Stress and illness stimulate our bodies to release "protective" hormones that in turn stimulate the release of stored glucose in the liver. This extra glucose serves as an emergency fuel reserve to help fight off disease-causing germs or to help react to a stressful episode. That response may be okay for people without diabetes, but for those with diabetes, it can be harmful. In Chapter 5 you'll learn how to cope with stress, and elsewhere in this book learn how to modify your diet, exercise, and medication when you are sick.

Low Blood Glucose

If blood glucose levels drop below normal, you may sometimes feel the effects. You may feel irritable, flaky, sweaty, headachy, or just plain "out of sorts." Or, you may not notice anything, but someone else recognizes a change in you. If your blood glucose levels continue to fall and you don't react, someone else will have to treat your condition.

When you feel symptoms that indicate low blood glucose, or when someone says you are acting strangely, eat something that contains sugar. Raisins, hard candy, or orange juice are all good choices if your schedule has been thrown off by travel or heavy traffic and you have missed or delayed a scheduled meal.

The best way to avoid low blood sugar episodes is to stick with your diabetes management plan: eat your meals and snacks according to schedule, exercise when you have planned, take your medication as prescribed, and check your blood glucose levels often.

Although it's important to know the symptoms and treatments for low blood glucose, most people with Type 2 non-insulin-dependent diabetes rarely have to worry about low blood glucose attacks. However, your risks increase if you take an oral hypoglycemic agent or inject insulin.

High Blood Glucose

If blood glucose levels stay elevated—above your normal range—for an extended time, there is a greatly increased risk for developing the complications associated with diabetes. Too much blood glucose over the years can damage the heart, blood vessels, nervous system, eyes, kidneys, and most other organs.

A brief episode of high blood glucose can make you feel good, similar to the feeling after a big meal. However, as we all know, eating a lot at one sitting can also make you feel fatigued, drowsy, and washed out. After a big meal you can expect an above-normal blood glucose measurement. Interestingly, the blood fat content would also be above normal if you measured it.

A big meal a couple times a week will send blood glucose levels up steadily. Of course, waistlines will also grow if the routine continues. Weight gain and high blood sugar readings day after day may cause low feelings, even depression. Some people will try to relieve their depression by eating another big meal, causing a vicious cycle that would be a nemesis for us all.

The risks associated with prolonged periods of high blood glucose can be great. For instance, if blood glucose levels remain above normal or even moderately high for an extended time, the extra glucose can damage nerves, resulting in the complication called diabetic neuropathy. This painful condition often affects the feet and legs.

Furthermore, prolonged periods of above-normal blood glucose in men can lead to impotence because of damage to the nerves or the blood vessels in the penis. In women, prolonged periods of above-normal blood glucose may result in an inability to reach sexual climax.

Both small and large blood vessels can be damaged by long periods of exposure to high blood glucose. The small blood vessels of the eyes are most often affected, leading to diabetic retinopathy, loss of visual acuity, and sometimes even blindness.

Blood vessels in the kidneys may also be damaged, and excess blood glucose is known to damage the large blood vessels, which can lead to heart disease, strokes, and circulation problems.

Finally, high blood glucose levels can speed up the aging process by accelerating such age-related problems as cataract formation and stiffening of the joints and skin. All of these complications are avoidable, however, if people stick to their diabetes management plans and work to keep their blood glucose within normal ranges.

CHAPTER 5

Your Emotions and Diabetes

EMOTIONS PLAY A KEY ROLE in a life with diabetes. In fact, they may be instrumental in making good choices for keeping your diabetes in tight control. It all starts with how you feel about the disease. This can determine the success of your management plan.

Your feelings about diabetes likely will change over the years, and not always predictably. When you were first diagnosed, were you angry? Depressed? Maybe you felt guilt for some reason. These feelings are natural and many people experience them.

Immediately after diagnosis and a little beyond, it is okay to feel that life dealt you a bad hand. But remember the words of the famous author, Robert Louis Stevenson: "Life is not a matter of having good cards, but of playing a poor hand well."

If you were down at first, the curative effects of time, support from friends, family, and health care professionals, and your own innate strength all will help you move beyond any initial anger and depression and get on with your life. With diabetes and its many choices and new and healthy tasks it requires, you can turn your situation into a plus. Use your health challenge to develop a positive, strengthened lifestyle.

Unfortunately, emotions, like blood glucose, do not remain steady. There will be days that you feel up and days you feel down. But that's true for everyone. No matter who you are, there are things in life that cause good feelings and things that cause something less. And then there are times that no matter how hard you work, nothing seems to go right. It's hard not to feel defeated, depressed, or distraught. We haven't even mentioned what others do, or don't do, that affect our feelings and actions.

All of these factors can add up to stress. Some stress you create yourself. Some stress comes from friends, family, and even strangers. Diabetes can also cause stress. Who knows? Some stress may even be created by the health professionals working to help you control your diabetes.

Bear in mind, however, that a little stress can be good. It can give that extra push all of us need to get moving and keep moving. Too much stress, though, can create major problems.

First, a large amount of stress can send blood glucose levels soaring. That's the body's natural response, a carryover from the early days when humans needed the "fight or flight" response to stay alive.

Second, a moderate to large amount of stress can affect our emotions. The result may be anxiety, panic, or sometimes immobilizing depression. When emotions are upset that much, you can bet that blood glucose control, and even an entire diabetes management plan, will likely be compromised.

So, what can you do? Stress is present to some extent in everyone's life. Since we can't avoid all sources of emotional stress, here are some tips for handling it:

LEARN TO STAY COOL when you know you are going to be in stressful situations (like when you are preparing for a discussion about room cleanliness with your favorite teenager).

RECOGNIZE THAT CERTAIN EVENTS ARE BOUND TO CREATE SOME STRESS—retirement, moving to a new house, planning a wedding. Anticipating the possibility that an event will cause stress will allow you time to come to grips with the situation. It's the unanticipated and uncontrollable sources of stress that are the most troublesome.

LEARN HOW TO COPE WITH STRESS when it does occur. Read on to learn how to recognize stress triggers, how to react, and what symptoms to look for.

Learning about Stress

One of the best ways to cope with stress is to learn how to relax. Everyone relaxes differently. What works for your spouse or friend may not work for you, but here we present some ideas.

CONSIDER CHECKING OUT SOME BOOKS at the library regarding relaxation techniques, stress modification, or meditation. Choose whatever books catch your eye, then do a little research on your own.

VIDEO RENTAL STORES may also be a research source. Many have tapes on meditation, relaxation, yoga, and biofeedback.

MANY COMMUNITY CENTERS AND HOSPITALS offer stress management courses. Check them out and take advantage of any learning opportunities.

Coping Strategies

MEDITATION: One of the oldest approaches to relaxation, meditation is a tradition in many religions that is described as the other side of prayer. In prayer, you speak; in meditation, you listen. Meditation takes time and should be done in a quiet, calm place. Sit silently and look inward at your thoughts and feelings. You don't need a mountaintop for meditation, you can do it in the privacy of your home or office, outdoors, or even on a coffee break.

Meditation has been shown to improve a number of the physical signs of stress, lowering pulse rates and blood pressure. Meditation has also been shown to help some people with Type 2 diabetes lower their blood glucose. You may not be able to get this effect immediately, but by practicing meditation, you will learn to relax your body and calm emotions.

IMAGING: This is a method of relaxation in which you create scenes in your mind that are soothing and pleasant for you. Once you learn the technique, you will be able to sit in your favorite chair, close your eyes, and create an image of yourself sitting on a sun-drenched beach, near a sparkling waterfall, or in a windswept field of flowers. In effect, you create a mini-vacation in your mind. And your emotional response to this freedom will be both relaxing and refreshing.

BIOFEEDBACK: This is a more scientific, organized approach to relaxation. It focuses on relaxing tense muscles using feedback equipment to tell you when you have succeeded. You learn to relax muscles by thinking "soothing" thoughts. You learn what your personal "soothing" messages are and how to make them work for you. Once mastered, you can use it whenever you feel yourself tensing up. You can also learn to aim relaxing messages at specific muscles. In some studies, up to 85 percent of the people with Type 2 diabetes successfully used biofeedback techniques to reduce stress-related high blood glucose levels.

From Morton's Journal

At first, I was very angry about the fact that I was diagnosed as having diabetes. It came at a bad time. I had just retired, and I was attempting to deal with this major change in my life. I had just moved to a new location and was trying to adjust to a radically new lifestyle. According to the experts, these two changes in life are among the top stress-producers. Then along came diabetes, which required even more lifestyle changes.

Adjusting to the move was a lot easier than adjusting to retirement. At first, I relaxed and enjoyed the palm trees and balmy weather. But, after a while (about 9 months) that became a bore. At my spouse's suggestion (other than get out of the house and do something), I went to the local volunteer center and offered my services. It was a revelation to me that so many opportunities for meaningful volunteer work were available. I enlisted and now find that I hardly have time to laze by the pool for extended periods. I find that I am much more relaxed, even though my body (and my mind) are working quite hard.

Having meaningful work (albeit without pay) certainly does put a positive accent on life and reduces the effects of stress caused by retirement, moving, the aging process, and most recently, the diagnosis of diabetes.

ACUPUNCTURE: Many people go to an acupuncturist for relaxation "tune-ups" that are reported to last several weeks to months.

PHYSICAL ACTIVITY: Taking a brisk walk in the early morning or the cool night air when we are upset is an age-old remedy for coping with stress. With exercise, you can concentrate on the physical activity and forget about troubling things. It's not escapism, it's just a way of coping with stress. And, it works.

Plus, being physically active tones muscles and builds blood vessels and lung heart capacity. Exercise also boosts the body's secretion of feel-good hormones. And when you feel good emotionally, you are more able to cope with life's stresses.

ATTITUDE ADJUSTMENT: In addition to coping with stress, one of the great challenges of diabetes is adopting and retaining a positive attitude. Most people have trouble seeing anything positive about diabetes immediately after being diagnosed with the chronic disease.

After some time passes, however, many see that life with diabetes is not so bad. In fact, it may be very good. If you think about it, the recommendations for managing diabetes are the same as those recommended for anyone who wants a long, healthy, and productive life:

People with diabetes should lose extra weight and keep it off. So should most Americans (most of whom are overweight).

People with diabetes need to eat a well balanced diet with lots of vegetables, grains, fruits, and vitamins and minerals and limited amounts of animal fat, sugar, and salt. So should most Americans (many of whom are at risk for heart disease, cancer, and stroke).

People with diabetes need to build physical activity and exercise into their daily life. So should most Americans (for whom the term "couch potato" was succinctly stated).

There may be a temptation to feel sorry for yourself. But, as you learn the facts about diabetes and the choices available to manage it, our hope is that you'll not only accept the diabetes, but find it gives you an advantage. Diabetes certainly provides a new motivation for health management, and you have an opportunity to take charge of both your diabetes and a healthier lifestyle.

Again, a person's attitude toward diabetes and life is a key to success. With a positive attitude, you'll make health-promoting choices that provide all the energy you need to live a healthy and productive life.

At the same time, don't feel tempted to ignore diabetes just because you start to feel well. Diabetes won't go away and it won't treat itself. Diabetes requires a consistent daily management program—eating plan, exercise program, blood glucose testing, and medication.

Some readers may not have any signs, symptoms, or complications of diabetes, other than the high blood glucose measurement reported at their doctor's office. But, they should realize that if they don't take care of their diabetes today, they greatly increase the risk of suffering serious complications in the future.

If you have trouble accepting your diagnosis, you run the risk of short-changing yourself for the future. You have the power to take control of your diabetes. In conclusion:

Diabetes is permanent and will cause you to change some aspects of your life;

You have the major responsibility for controlling the disease, but your actions can and will improve your diabetes and general health;

You will have to make informed and intelligent choices about meals and snacks and also build more physical activity into your life, but family, friends, and your diabetes team are available for support;

You will also be asked to make choices about monitoring your body's status—blood glucose, eyes, skin, feet, circulation, and digestion. This will require being watched more closely and more often by health professionals;

Finally, continual changes in your lifestyle may be needed to fine-tune your health.

People can accept or reject these facts as they wish. However, those who do accept the realities of the disease are better able to take a positive approach and stay on target in managing diabetes and their lives. Take the opportunity to turn what some consider a negative into a big plus.

CHAPTER 6

Food:
It's Your Choice

WHAT YOU EAT, how much you eat, and when you eat are three of the most important aspects of controlling diabetes. In fact, by not following a proper eating plan, all other efforts to control diabetes may be in vain.

In diabetes management, food is more important than exercise; it is more important than medication; and it is more important than blood glucose monitoring. Simply put, it is the most important element in your management program.

It goes without saying that the body can't function properly without food. The digestive system converts food into glucose, which is used as fuel (energy) to keep organs running smoothly, build tissue and bone, and, simply, keep us alive.

Some food is digested and converted to glucose rapidly, like table sugar, which is a simple carbohydrate. Complex carbohydrate-containing food, such as whole wheat bread, takes longer to digest and be converted into glucose. The protein in a steak takes even longer to digest and be converted into glucose. Fat is the slowest of all nutrients to be digested and converted into glucose.

Without the right kind of food, in the right amounts, and at the right times, all other parts of a diabetes management program will fail. Too much food will cause weight gain and send blood glucose and blood fat levels soaring. It will also put a person at great risk for cardiovascular disease and the long-term complications of diabetes.

A Love Affair

Many people's lifelong love affair with food has contributed to the development of their diabetes. And it has also contributed greatly to those extra pounds too many people carry around.

Being overweight and inheriting the genetic defect that leads to the development of Type 2 diabetes are two of the major risk factors for this type of diabetes. Most readers have both of them, plus the third risk factor: being over 40 years of age.

We cannot do anything if we have inherited a gene that puts us at risk. Nor can we turn back the clock to stop the aging process. But we can control the foods we select and quantities we consume.

For most of us, our eating habits developed in childhood at the family kitchen table. We ate what was put in front of us or we went hungry. We could not, without incurring the wrath of our parents, refuse to eat what was on our plate. A clean plate was equated with being a model child.

When you polished off ever-increasing portions to help you grow big and strong, were you rewarded? Perhaps a second helping or some pie or cake? Maybe real ice cream, loaded with fat. Another common snack was whole milk and a handful of cookies or a big slice of rich, creamy chocolate cake.

Eating habits we learned at that kitchen table have stayed with most of us throughout our lives. Oh, perhaps they have been modified by the addition of convenience foods, microwaveable dinners, and fast food. But for many people, food is still a reward.

Oftentimes, though, the "reward" leads to extra inches in the waistline, thighs, arms, and elsewhere. If you have developed the habit of overeating and eating the wrong foods, it may be hard to change this lifelong pattern, but it is not impossible!

When you were first diagnosed with Type 2 diabetes, did your doctor tell you that you must lose those excess pounds to bring your blood glucose levels back down to your normal range? Your doctor might have told you that you need to get down to your "ideal" weight according to your age, height, and sex. Some people are told to go on a strict diet.

The problem is, many people try to diet—they even lose

weight—but in no time they return to their normal patterns of eating and their weight goes back up. So they try it again. And get the same results. This very discouraging pattern of weight loss and gain is called the yo-yo dieting syndrome.

If this has been your experience, don't despair. Scientists now agree that most weight-loss plans are useless. Most conventional weight-loss plans can't be followed for a long time and most demand that you lose lots of weight quickly. To be successful, you should consult a doctor or dietitian and:

Take it slowly!

Instead of trying to trim down to the body you had when you were 20 in a few weeks, try to take small steps to cut down your excess weight.

Small weight losses provide big benefits!

If, over a reasonable period, you lose just 10 or 20 pounds (or 10 percent of your body weight), you will still see significant improvements in blood glucose levels. Lose these pounds by making small reductions in the amounts of food you eat and by making better food choices. Try cutting down on high-fat, high-calorie foods and substitute them with tasty low-fat, high-fiber, lower-calorie ones.

Move it! Exercise plus a new lower calorie foodstyle will double your benefits.

The bottom line is that you need a new eating plan, not a diet. Your personal eating plan can be both satisfying and healthful. Here are the nutrition guidelines that can help.

Nutrition Guidelines

The American Diabetes Association (ADA) recently revised its nutrition guidelines for people with diabetes, based on current scientific nutrition and diabetes knowledge. The first nutrition guidelines were developed in 1986. These were somewhat rigid and restricted sugar, fat, and calories, based on eating plans developed for the "average" person with diabetes.

The new nutrition guidelines stress flexibility. Their many goals include:

• maintaining near-normal blood glucose levels;

- achieving optimal blood-fat levels;
- attaining a reasonable weight;
- preventing complications;
- improving overall health through optimal nutrition.

Your personal eating plan, grounded in these new rules, can be tailored to your lifestyle, not just to your diabetes.

If you take an oral hypoglycemic agent, or if you inject insulin, your meals and snacks need to be balanced with your medication and insulin action, your exercise and activity level, and your blood glucose levels. Whether or not you take diabetes medication, your eating plan needs to help you improve your control of blood glucose, blood pressure, and blood-fat (lipid) levels.

Current research suggests you should work on lowering your blood glucose and blood fat levels and expect to lose only small amounts of weight in small amounts of time. This weight loss is achievable, not by following a strict low-calorie diet, but by making better food choices.

In your new eating plan, you can:
- select foods that are low in saturated fat and calories;
- spread your meals from the traditional three squares a day to the "grazing" approach of six or more small meals throughout the day;
- cut down your calorie intake each day by 250 to 500 calories by reducing portion sizes.

It's also a great help to add an extra 10 or 15 minutes of exercise activities to your daily schedule.

If you are interested in having your diabetes eating plan fit the ADA nutrition guidelines, the first step should be to consult with your doctor. Your doctor will evaluate your current level of control and then refer you to a dietitian who can develop an eating plan that fits you to a T.

Here are some key points in the ADA's guidelines:

PROTEIN: 10 to 20 percent of your daily calorie intake should be from protein sources, either plant or meat sources. People with kidney disease (diabetic nephropathy), should limit their protein intake to 10 percent or less of total daily calories.

TOTAL FAT: Recommended daily amounts of fat differ, depending on whether you are at your "ideal" weight, overweight, or have high blood fat (cholesterol) levels. There are also restrictions on the types of fat you should eat and whether the fat should be saturated, polyunsaturated, or monounsaturated.

Interestingly, everyone needs some fat in their daily eating plan, so choose this with care. Dietary fat is required for growth and stored as an emergency source of energy. For most adults, scientists now recommend that 30 percent of your daily calories come from fat, with up to 10 percent from polyunsaturated fat, and less than 10 percent from saturated fat.

Since fat is a concentrated source of calories, one of the best ways to reduce calories (and weight) is to reduce your intake of total fat, which works particularly well when you also increase your exercise. Read food labels and you'll find lots of low- and lower-fat options in the market.

If you have elevated levels of blood fats, such as cholesterol or triglycerides, your doctor and dietitian may recommend that you lower your total fat intake and increase the percentage of mono-unsaturated fat intake to 20 percent of total calories, while reducing your intake of saturated or polyunsaturated types of fat.

CARBOHYDRATES AND SWEETENERS: Perhaps the best news in the new nutrition guidelines is, "Scientific evidence has shown that the use of sucrose (table sugar) as part of the meal plan does not impair blood glucose control in individuals with Type 1 or Type 2 diabetes."

Wait! Before you rush out and eat a triple scoop of mint-chocolate chip ice cream, take another look at this statement.

What the experts are saying is that sugar may be part of a well balanced meal that contains protein, fat, and carbohydrates. A high-sugar food should not be eaten alone as a snack because it can send blood glucose levels soaring. As part of a well balanced meal, however, sugar (in place of other carbohydrates) does not have this effect on post-meal blood glucose levels.

The same experts also report that sugar and sugar-containing foods must be substituted for other carbohydrates in your eating plan, not simply added to an already balanced meal.

Your individualized eating plan should give priority to total amounts of carbohydrate, rather than sources of that carbohydrate. The guidelines also state that other nutritive sweeteners (corn syrup, fruit juice, molasses, honey, dextrose, and maltose) do not have any significant advantage or disadvantage over simple sugar in terms of calories or blood glucose response. Fructose, however, may offer some advantages as a sweetener, but it has the potential for creating unwanted side effects. Natural sources of fructose, such as fruits and vegetables, are the best choices.

FIBER: Dietary fiber intake of 20 to 35 grams per day from a variety of food sources is recommended for all adults, including those with diabetes. The effect of dietary fiber on blood glucose control, according to the ADA guidelines, is probably insignificant.

SODIUM: The guidelines recommend that sodium restrictions be the same for people with diabetes as for the general population—no more than 3,000 milligrams per day. For people with mild to moderate hypertension (high blood pressure), 2,400 milligrams per day or less is recommended.

ALCOHOL: Under normal circumstances blood glucose control will not be affected by moderate use of alcohol, when diabetes is well controlled. Keep in mind, however, that alcohol may strengthen the hypoglycemic action of insulin, possibly leading to low blood glucose levels. If you inject insulin, your dosage may need to be adjusted. Talk to your doctor about this.

Also, if you inject insulin, you should limit yourself to two alcoholic drinks a day. A typical "drink" is 12 ounces of beer, 4 ounces of wine, or 1 1/2 ounces of liquor. When possible, choose light beers and dry wines because they have fewer calories. Watch out for sugary drinks, like wine coolers, and mixed drinks made with regular soda pop or juice.

If you are working to control your weight, remember that alcoholic beverages contain "empty" calories that must be counted in your daily total but do not provide any nutritional value.

From Morton's Journal

I hate to diet. I love to eat. I like to cook. I enjoy eating good foods. Because of my likes and dislikes, I have overdone eating. And, over the years, this habit has translated into extra pounds. But I hate diets. I've tried a dozen of them ranging from grapefruit and water to using appetite-suppressing medications. None worked.

Because of my work as a medical writer, I read all about the hazards of fats, sugars, and salt. Using my brain instead of my taste-buds, I made an effort to cut down on my intake of fats, sugars, and salt. In fact, at our house table sugar and salt are banned from the dining room and kitchen.

I've added fish and poultry to the menu, and reduced the number of times a week we eat beef, lamb, and pork. Fresh vegetables and fruits are always regular visitors to our daily menu. What I didn't do (until I attended a diabetes class) was cut down on the amount of food—the portion size—on my plate.

One of the most important things in my dietary adventures was the discovery of what should be a healthy portion size. This discovery took place during a lecture I attended as part of the diabetes management course offered at Sarasota Memorial Hospital by the Diabetes Treatment Services. After listening to the nutrition expert explain what "exchanges" were, and how to calculate calories and carbohydrates, we students were shown food models that were sized to "healthy portions." How small they were. How much larger were my usual portions.

Kicking Off Your Eating Plan

Remember, the most "freedom" in meal planning can be yours if your diabetes is in good control. If you are having control challenges, you may need a more rigid approach initially. Once you maintain good control, however, you can be more flexible with your eating plan food choices.

If you have recently been diagnosed with Type 2 diabetes, your doctor may recommend that you follow a "kickoff" eating plan. This plan requires that you temporarily reduce your intake of carbohydrates to less than 40 percent of your daily total. As your blood glucose levels drop into the normal range, you may be able to increase your total carbohydrate intake.

Again, be sure to check with your doctor before starting any eating plan. Furthermore, if you are taking medication to treat high blood pressure, these recommendations may not be right for you.

Some newly diagnosed people who are overweight find that it is easier to abstain completely from eating for a time than it is to try to eat very small portions. For these people, there is a "kickoff" eating plan built around a three-day fast. Use caution, though; this approach needs to be supervised by a member of your diabetes health care team and must never be done without medical support.

During a three-day fast you do not eat any food, although you may drink water. Before and during the fast, frequent blood glucose measurements (a minimum of four times a day) are needed and should be recorded in a diary or log.

The fast may not work for everyone. But, if you respond to the fast, you'll note that your blood glucose levels drop from above-normal into the normal range, usually without any diabetes medication.

After the three-day fast, you'll begin to eat food again, but on a reduced-calorie eating plan. The amount of calories allowed on the plan will be determined by your doctor, with your consent.

Initially, the eating plan will be relatively low in carbohydrate content, about 40 percent. Because of this restriction on carbohydrates, you'll probably eat more fat than you normally would, and certainly more fat than you'll eat when you normalize your blood glucose levels. Be extra careful about the type of fat you eat. Avoid foods that are high in saturated fats, such as meat, and choose foods that contain monounsaturated fats and polyunsaturated fats, such as olive oil or vegetable oils.

Although an extended high-fat diet is known to increase the risks of heart disease, this particular plan is intended to be a short-term one—designed to quickly bring your blood glucose levels down into the normal range. It is also a good start for losing excess pounds.

Don't set unrealistic goals, however. For instance, if you think you can't follow a 1,200-calorie-a-day eating plan, tell your doctor in advance. You may need to start at a high calorie intake and spread your weight loss over a greater period. Do what works for you.

After a three-day fast, you'll probably find that you won't be as hungry and won't need as much food to satisfy your hunger. That's because your stomach, literally, shrinks during the three days. By making wise food choices, you'll find it easier to reduce your calorie intake.

Your Personal Eating Plan

Your diabetes eating plan should be designed specifically for you by a dietitian and you should be able to follow it comfortably every day. With time, however, your lifestyle and body changes, so your eating plan will also need to change.

No one diabetes eating plan is effective for everyone. Each meal in the plan must be tailored to the individual, so planning is the key.

Keep in mind that your eating plan needs are quite different than the needs of someone with Type 1 diabetes. Also, eating plans for an overweight or underweight person will differ from that for a person at their ideal weight.

Perhaps the best advice for most overweight people with Type 2 diabetes is to work on establishing a new eating lifestyle—one that features moderate to small portions of tasty foods prepared in a healthful way. Add to this some daily exercise and your new healthier lifestyle is underway.

There are a variety of ways to approach an eating plan. The most popular options are outlined below. You'll see that each has specific benefits and drawbacks. Review the options, talk with your dietitian about specifics, then pick a comfortable method for you, one that will help you maintain good diabetes control.

The Exchange System

The exchange system is the one of most popular and widely used systems. It is supported by the American Diabetes Association. The exchange system groups foods into size categories, with measured portions of approximately the same nutritional value. Food choices within the same group can be exchanged with, or substituted for, other foods in the same category. Many people use exchange food groups that are defined as Starch/Breads, Meat/Meat Substitutes, Vegetables, Fruits, Milk, and Fat.

Others are learning the newly revised exchange system, which defines three main categories of food groups: Carbohydrate, Meat and Meat Substitute, and Fat. The Carbohydrate group includes vegetables, fruit, and milk, in addition to starch foods and other carbohydrates. The Meat and Meat Substitute group lists foods according to their fat content: very lean, lean, medium-fat, and high-fat. And the Fat group is divided according to the main type of fat in foods: monounsaturated, polyunsaturated, and saturated.

The exchange system is particularly useful to people who like structure and specific instructions on how to make food choices. Unfortunately, the system is a bit difficult to learn at first. Much of the nutrition information needs to be memorized, so the system may seem overwhelming to some.

The ADA has developed a "Healthy Food Choices" program, based on the exchange program, to help simplify eating plans using the exchange system.

Carbohydrate Counting

This system of meal planning allows you to calculate the amount of carbohydrates you eat at each meal. This way you can maintain consistency in carbohydrate intake from day to day, which is a great plus for a person with Type 2 diabetes. Another advantage of this carbohydrate counting is that it allows you to eat any kind of carbohydrate (within your quota for the meal) whether that carbohydrate is simple (such as sugar) or complex (when it comes from whole wheat bread).

To start this system, you need to work out your meal quotas with a dietitian on your diabetes health care team. Once you have these (either measured in grams or units), you can then plan your meals. You will need to learn portion sizes (as you do with other meal planning systems) and then determine the carbohydrate content of these portions. Reading labels on prepared foods, such as in cans and frozen packages, makes this a bit easier. For fresh foods, you will have to consult your nutrition books. Good news on this front, though, for many fresh foods are now carrying labels that provide information concerning portion size, calorie, carbohydrate, fat, and protein content.

You'll also have to calculate the amount of soluble fiber in the foods you eat. Such fiber is considered a carbohydrate, but since it is not fully or rapidly digested, you will have to deduct fiber-carbohydrate from your mealtime quota.

Carbohydrate counting is of particular value to people who are injecting insulin, because the system allows them to be more precise in the dosage of insulin they will need to "cover" the carbohydrate content of a meal.

Although this system enables you to calculate your carbohydrate intake and maintain control of your intake, you still have to keep in mind that your meals require a healthy balance of nutrients. You can't eat just carbohydrate-containing foods. Your body also needs protein, fat, vitamins, and minerals. When you do your meal planning, you will also have to calculate the amount (and type) of protein and fat you will be having, and the total amount of essential vitamins and minerals. Your dietitian can be of great help to you in planning a meal program that assures you that your food intake is well balanced.

Calorie/Fat Counting System

The calorie/fat counting system seems best for people who have a knack for working with numbers and want flexibility in food choices. The system requires you to "count" the number of calories and the grams of fat in all the food for each meal and to stay within a set quota established for the weight-loss or maintenance eating plan.

On the down side, this system does not take into account carbohydrates, protein, fiber, or vitamins and minerals. Also, it does not cover the scheduling of meals and snacks or the particular composition of those meals. Because of these limitations, the system is most useful during a weight-loss period, but is not well suited for the long term.

The Point System

The point system is a structured, simplified method for counting calories and specific nutrient contents. For example, 75 calories is equal to one calorie point; two or three grams of fat are equal to one fat point. The eating plan establishes point quotas for both calories and nutrients.

If you use this plan, you must make food choices based on point quotas. This is fairly easy to learn and provides flexibility in making food choices. It does, however, require calculating various point values of food choices and recording points or food choices in a diary or log.

Preparing individualized eating plans based on the point system is a significant challenge for dietitians.

Following the system, however, does give the person with Type 2 diabetes an excellent opportunity to learn about nutrition requirements and dietary guidelines.

The Food Pyramid

The Food Pyramid is the current basic dietary recommendation for all Americans. It replaces the four basic food groups that you probably learned about in grammar school. Now, daily serving guidelines are based on their location in a pyramid. As you can see from the following illustration, fats, oils, and sweets are at the top of the pyramid. Their position means we should consume only small quantities of these in proportion to the other food groups in the pyramid.

The Food Pyramid

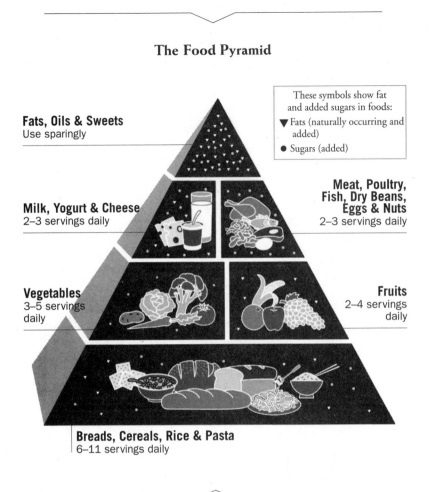

Fats, Oils & Sweets
Use sparingly

These symbols show fat and added sugars in foods:
▼ Fats (naturally occurring and added)
● Sugars (added)

Milk, Yogurt & Cheese
2–3 servings daily

Meat, Poultry, Fish, Dry Beans, Eggs & Nuts
2–3 servings daily

Vegetables
3–5 servings daily

Fruits
2–4 servings daily

Breads, Cereals, Rice & Pasta
6–11 servings daily

Meat, poultry, dry beans, eggs, and nuts, and milk, yogurt, and cheese are next down in the pyramid. Fruits, vegetables, bread, cereal, rice, and pasta make up the base, meaning the bulk of our daily calories should come from these sources.

The pyramid does not, however, provide specific meal-by-meal guidelines or the structure for people who need to know the nutrient composition of their meals and snacks.

Other Systems

Three systems—the high carbohydrate, high fiber (HCF) system, total available glucose (TAG) system, and glycemic index system—provide structured approaches to an eating plan for only the highly motivated. For most people, they are difficult to learn and do and can be extremely time consuming.

However, if you are inclined toward a scientific understanding of Type 2 diabetes, work with your doctor and nutritionist to understand how to use these systems.

From Morton's Journal

The nutritionist at the diabetes education course that I attended explained all of the different meal planning approaches. Although class members were taught to calculate exchanges, I was less interested in this method. I found it too constraining. I really didn't want to bother with calculations each time I sat down to eat. My diabetes educator supported my decision to follow a healthy food selection/preparation approach, particularly if I could restrain myself on portion size.

Since I never had a sweet tooth, I could avoid sugary snacks.

Since I banned salt from the table and from most cooking, I could restrict sodium intake.

Since I switched to artificial sweeteners, I could avoid excess sugar.

Since I added more poultry and fish to the home menu, I could cut down on fatty meats.

But I have to remind myself (constantly) to cut portion sizes, to leave some food on the plate (contrary to what my mother advised me), and to seriously reduce my visits to pizza parlors, burger joints, and seafood restaurants that serve fried calamari and other deep-fried delights. I reminded myself that I didn't have to totally give up these treats, but I did have to restrain myself (and do all the other things necessary to keep my blood glucose within the normal range).

How to Judge Portion Sizes

The first thing to know about eating plans is how to estimate portion sizes of both solids and liquids. At first, you should probably practice with measuring tools: cups, glasses, spoons, scales, and the like. But once you know the exact measures, you'll be able to estimate correct portion sizes when they are served.

These skills are important for making accurate visual estimations of food. Use measuring tools, like a scale, rather than trusting your eyes when you are trying new foods in your eating plan.

How to Figure Percentage of Calories From Fat

No matter what eating plan you choose, you will probably have to pay more attention to the nutrient information on food labels. You may be surprised by your findings. Seemingly "healthy" foods may have more fat or salt than you previously thought.

Percentage of calories from fat is one the most important measurements in meal planning. To calculate the percentage of total calories from fat in a given food product, multiply the grams of fat per serving by 9. (Each gram of fat contains 9 calories.) Divide this number by the total number of calories in each serving of the specific food. Multiply this number by 100 to convert it to a percentage.

For example, a food that contains 3 grams of fat per serving and 100 calories per serving would be calculated as follows:

3 grams of fat x 9 = 27 fat calories

27 divided by 100 (calories per serving) = 0.27

0.27 x 100 = 27% of the calories in a serving comes from fat

How to Read Food Labels

Food labels are required to contain the following information:
- Serving size
- Servings per container
- Information per serving: calories, calories from fat, total fat in grams, saturated fat in grams, cholesterol in milligrams, sodium in milligrams, total carbohydrate in grams, dietary fiber in grams, sugar in grams, and protein in grams

- All nutritional claims on food labels must comply with new, stricter requirements, which should make healthy shopping easier. For example:

Low calorie means 40 calories or less per serving.
Low fat means 3 grams of fat or less per serving.
Low cholesterol means 20 milligrams or less per serving.
Sugar-free means the product contains less than 0.5 grams of sugar per serving.

Almost all packaged foods list their ingredients on the label, in order, according to their weight in the product. So, the first ingredient is the one in the greatest quantity in the product.

Shopping and Cooking for an Eating Plan
Here are some tips to accommodate your eating plan:
- Make a list of foods that you need to buy. Do your best to stick to the list and avoid impulse buying.
- Avoid the candy, cookie, and high-fat snacks aisles. Although you may find some low-fat packaged snacks, think first of fresh, crunchy vegetables.
- Buy fresh fruits and vegetables when possible.
- Select reduced- or low-fat dairy products such as skim milk and fat-free cheese.
- Select poultry and fish as your primary protein sources.
- Look for low-fat and fat-free cold cuts in the deli. Double-check the labels to make sure they are indeed low fat.
- Use beans, pasta, rice, and vegetables for inexpensive, healthful main dishes.
- Prepare foods by broiling, roasting, baking, boiling, or steaming, instead of frying.
- Choose nonstick vegetable oil spray if you plan to sauté or pan fry.
- Select whipped or reduced-calorie vegetable margarines instead of butter.
- Select plain, nonfat yogurt as a substitute for sour cream in recipes and as a topping.

- Select an egg substitute or use egg whites only for breakfast or in recipes.
- Choose artificial sweeteners for table and cooking use.

Here's our list of tips for a more healthful cooking style. Note that some of these bear repeating:
- Use a nonstick vegetable spray to sauté or pan fry.
- Bake, broil, roast, steam, or grill; don't fry.
- Use whipped or reduced-calorie vegetable margarines when you must add fat to foods.
- Reduce the fat in recipes by identifying acceptable ingredient substitutions.
- Use only nonfat or reduced-fat dairy products (milk, yogurt, or cheese).
- Use two egg whites instead of one whole egg in recipes. Eliminating yolks cuts out the cholesterol.

To decrease the amount of sugar in cooking:
- Use alternative sweeteners like saccharin, aspartame (Nutra-Sweet), or acesulfame-K (Sunette) at the table and in recipes. Use products containing these sweeteners instead of those sweetened with table sugar or corn syrup.
- Cut the amount of sugar in recipes to no more than one teaspoon per serving, or use a sugar substitute.
- Omit sugar-containing glazes or icing on baked goods.
- Use recipes from cookbooks designed for people with diabetes. (See the list at the end of this chapter.)

To decrease sodium in your eating plan:
- Use low-sodium or nonsalt herb mixtures instead of regular salt at the table and in recipes.
- Select only frozen dinners that contain less than 800 milligrams of sodium and less than 30 percent of calories from fat.
- Substitute for or avoid high-sodium foods such as processed meats, catsup, meat tenderizers, soy sauce, bouillon, barbecue sauce, steak sauce, and canned or convenience foods (such as soup mixes, snack foods, regular canned soups, and

regular peanut butter). Many of these products are available in low-sodium versions, so be sure to read the labels.

Eating Plan for When You're on the Road
When you travel:
- Stock a small cooler with a container of cold water, cans of fruit juice, or sugar-free beverages.
- Pack lean chicken or turkey breast slices in plastic bags for your cooler and a loaf of whole grain bread for quick sandwiches when you need them.
- Take along fresh fruit and pack ready-to-eat fresh vegetables in plastics bags in your cooler.
- Order special meals in advance. Most airlines, railroads, and cruise lines now feature low-calorie, low-fat, low-sugar cuisines. If special meals are not available, choose the lowest calorie and fat options on the menu, then supplement your meal with one of your own snacks.

Quick Tips for Eating Out
- Stay away from burgers, fries, and other high-fat items. Even fast-food outlets now offer healthier selections.
- Eat raw vegetables or fruit as appetizers.
- Choose high-fiber, whole grain breads and rolls; avoid croissants and biscuits.
- Select lean cuts of meat, fish, or poultry. Order your protein course broiled, baked, roasted, or grilled.
- Avoid dishes that include gravies or thick sauces.
- Request a luncheon-sized portion instead of a full dinner portion.
- Order salad with dressing on the side. Choose your dressings carefully to fit your eating plan.

Cookbooks for Your Eating Plan Bookshelf

Here's a short list of excellent cookbooks for anyone wanting to prepare healthy meals, diabetes or not:

ADA Family Cookbook—The American Tradition Family Cookbook (Volume IV), Prentice Hall Press, New York, 1991. May be ordered from the American Diabetes Association.

All-American Low-Fat & No-Fat Meals in Minutes, second edition, Chronimed Publishing, Minneapolis, 1997.

The Carbohydrate Counting Cookbook, Chronimed Publishing, Minneapolis, 1998.

Cooking Light Annual Cookbook, Oxmoor House, Birmingham, AL, published annually.

Diabetic Low-Fat & No-Fat Meals in Minutes, Chronimed Publishing, Minneapolis, 1996.

Jane Brody's Good Food Cookbook, W.W. Norton and Co., New York, 1985.

The USCD Healthy Diet for Diabetes, Houghton Mifflin Co., Boston, 1990.

CHAPTER 7

Exercise:
The Options are Plentiful

WHEN YOU HEAR the word *exercise,* what do you think of? A spirited game of tennis? Challenging 2-mile run? Fast-paced aerobics? Fortunately, exercise has much more broader applications. Sure, swimming several laps or taking a 30-minute walk can do wonders for your body, mental state, and diabetes. But so can exercise in the form of mowing the lawn or cleaning the house. Here are some of the benefits of exercise.

- Improves your blood glucose control, keeping levels in the normal range, and it reduces the risks of developing diabetes-related complications.
- Reduces blood fat levels and the risks for heart attacks and strokes.
- Contributes to weight loss (with the help of a diet emphasizing reduced fat and calories) and helps keep weight off.
- Improves muscle tone and flexibility.
- Reduces reactions to stress.
- Helps you feel better emotionally. And when you feel good, your energy levels increase, too.
- Reduces a woman's risks for developing osteoporosis after menopause (in combination with a calcium-rich diet).
- Can slow the aging process by toning muscles, strengthening bones, and making joints flexible.
- May increase your life span.

That's not a bad list of benefits from a single source.

These benefits are yours from any number of kinds of exercise or physical activity. The choices are yours.

If you think you're too old to begin some sort of exercise program, forget it. You are also never too overweight or too burdened by physical limitations to exercise. Special exercise programs can be designed for the elderly, overweight, or physically challenged person.

It all starts with making a commitment to an exercise program. If you need some prompting, just review the previous list of benefits.

There are plenty of excuses not to exercise: I'm too tired. Too busy. Bored by exercise. Not convinced it will work. Can't afford to join a health club or buy special equipment or clothing.

Sound familiar? Almost all of us have used one of these excuses or a variation at one time or another. But we'd like you to declare today as the day you put excuses aside and consider the many changes that have occurred in the approach to exercise.

We alluded to the most important change at the beginning of this chapter: Researchers say you can get the same positive benefits of exercise if you engage in all sorts of physical activity. Things like lawnwork, walking to the store, or steady housework all qualify as physical activity. Doing something three or four times a day for 10 minutes each session, each and every day, is just as beneficial as a half-hour workout at the gym.

Of course, you can opt for more formal exercise such as cycling, brisk walking, swimming, tennis, or aerobics. Just make sure to do it at least 30 minutes (plus warm-up and cool-down time) every other day. Or you can chose to do intense exercise—cycling for one hour four times a week, walking at four to five miles an hour for 45 minutes five times a week, for instance.

Today we can choose any one of these approaches to exercise. That's new. A few years ago we believed all exercise programs had to be formal and rigid. Before you exercise your exercise options, however, first check with your doctor. Have a checkup and get an evaluation of your physical status. Your doctor can then recommend which exercise program may be best for you. This is particularly important if you have any complications of diabetes.

After you get the go-ahead from the doctor, proceed very slowly at first with your choice of exercise programs. We emphasize slowly because if you are like most adults, you have not done much exercise in a number of years—quite possibly since your school days.

Exercise goals are another necessity. What do you want to achieve by becoming more physically active? Do you want to lose 20 pounds? If so, remember that you'll also have to follow an eating plan with reduced-fat and reduced-calorie foods. Exercise alone won't do it!

One more consideration: It has taken most people a long time to add 20 extra pounds, so they shouldn't expect to lose them overnight, or even in a few weeks. Set a realistic goal of losing 1 or 1 1/2 pounds each week. Such a goal is achievable, and it will ensure that your program has a chance to succeed. It will also increase the possibility of keeping the weight off once you lose it.

You can choose the types and approaches to exercise that fit your lifestyle best:

If you add physical activity to your life in the form of 10-minute sessions, three to four times each day, you should determine just what those activities will be and when you will do them. Use an activity diary or calendar to schedule your mini-exercise sessions and keep track of your progress.

If you choose a more formal approach to exercise, equip yourself with the necessary shoes, clothing, and equipment. Again, note on a calendar when you are going to exercise and stick with it.

A formal exercise program takes about 50 minutes every other day. Start with 10 minutes to warm up with stretching and bending exercises. Then do the formal exercise for 25 to 30 minutes. After that, take another 10 minutes to cool down with more stretching and bending exercises. To gain all the benefits, schedule your formal exercise for at least every other day.

You might want to join a health club. That choice will require some commuting time and paying membership fees, which may be a burden for some. For others, though, a financial commitment is a great motivator: "I paid for it, so I'd better do it."

If at all possible, get a friend or family member as a partner in your exercise program. Partners not only provide companionship, but they can also motivate. Make a commitment to each other to stick with the exercise program.

Whatever your exercise choice, be sure it is something you enjoy. Avoid boredom by building variety into your program. It helps to have a few alternative exercise options. For instance, if it's too hot to walk, go swimming. Or if you don't feel like tennis, play basketball.

And by all means, reward yourself when you achieve an exercise goal. Buy some new clothes or treat yourself to a play or concert. Just don't reward yourself with a 1000-calorie slice of chocolate cake!

From Morton's Journal

Exercise. What a bore! It takes a real mental effort on my part to decide to exercise. It's really mind over matter, particularly when I know I should be doing 30 to 40 minutes of exercise three or four times a week. When I was younger...much younger, I had gotten into the habit of jogging (before it was "in") at least three miles a day every other day. Then I hurt my ankle, and there went that habit out the window.

It seems that the decision to exercise has become harder with each passing year. Although I find it easy and enjoyable to go for a swim, particularly on a hot day, I really consider swimming a recreation, not exercise.

Compounding my problem with exercise is the fact that I am surrounded by active neighbors (many seniors, some younger) who constantly get up at the crack of dawn to walk mile upon mile on our uncrowded streets, or bike through the neighborhood greeting everyone as if they were the Good Humor man (or woman).

My exercise breakthrough came when a border collie named Rocky entered our family. His is lively and energetic and quite persuasive. He wants (and needs) to go for long walks at least three times a day. And since my wife is so busy with volunteer work (and her treadmill), the responsibility to take Rocky for walks falls upon my shoulders (and feet). So away we go, for 30 minutes of fast walking (with a few stops for sniffing and nature calls).

Rocky removed from me the responsibility of making a decision for exercise. A few woofs from him and we are off. And, although I am reluctant to admit it, the walking makes me feel better, both physically and mentally. And it's not bad, sniffing the smells of nature along with him. Plus, he's a great exercise companion.

No matter what type of exercise you choose, keep these three things in mind:

1. MONITOR YOUR BLOOD GLUCOSE MORE FREQUENTLY, particularly when you start an exercise program or switch to a new type of exercise. Check your blood glucose levels before and after each exercise session (and during long sessions of more than 30 minutes). See how exercise affects blood glucose levels. If your blood glucose levels are above or below your normal range, don't exercise unless you make the right modifications in your overall diabetes management program. This may mean eating a snack before exercising if your blood glucose levels are low, or adjusting your medication dosage if your levels are high.

2. KEEP TRACK OF YOUR PROGRESS. Use a diary or calendar to record what kind of exercise you did, at what intensity, and for how long. Check these records with your blood glucose measurements pre- and post-exercise, and with your weekly weight measurements. By using a diary you can document the benefits of your exercise program. If you are doing well, these positive results will be a great motivator. If things aren't going so well, these records will provide details you need to make appropriate changes.

3. LISTEN TO YOUR BODY. Don't exercise if it is too hot or too cold. Don't exercise if you don't feel well. Don't exercise if you have an illness. Don't exercise if you have an injury like a sprain or muscle strain. Take a day or two off if you have moderate to severe aches or pains. But make your "vacation" a short one. It's easy to get out of the exercise habit. Benefits disappear much more quickly than they accrue, so stick with it whenever you can.

Complications

If you have a diabetes-related complication, you can still choose an appropriate exercise program. But that program should be designed to fit your physical limitations and should never contribute to further harm. Here are some exercise tips if you have complications.

Neuropathy that Affects the Feet or Legs:

- Get a checkup from a podiatrist (foot doctor) as well as your diabetes doctor before you start any type of exercise.
- With your doctor's okay, choose an exercise that is non-weight-bearing, such as swimming or biking.
- Wear shoes and socks that provide the proper support and protection.
- Check your feet thoroughly every day before you exercise. Look for any problems, such as blisters, cuts, or swelling. If you detect a problem, do not exercise. Contact your foot doctor immediately for treatment.

Eye Problems:

- Get a checkup from your eye doctor in addition to one from your diabetes doctor before you start an exercise program.
- Choose exercises such as walking, low-impact aerobics, biking, or swimming. These do not jar or bounce your body, which may harm small blood vessels in the eyes.
- Avoid exercises such as weight training or aerobic gymnastics.

- Wear protective eyegear, if needed.
- If your vision changes while you are exercising, stop immediately. Contact your eye doctor about this problem before you resume exercising.

Heart and Kidney Problems:
- Be sure to get a checkup from all of your doctors before you start any exercise program. You should get specific instructions as to the type, frequency, and intensity of exercise you should do.
- With your doctor's okay, choose aerobic exercises that will strengthen your cardiovascular system. Do these exercises at a moderate intensity level, starting slowly, and gradually increasing the pace.
- Have your blood pressure checked regularly.
- Increase your fluid intake, if you have kidney problems, to prevent dehydration.

Age:
Some people consider age to be a barrier to exercise, or use it as an excuse not to exercise. Age, however, does not have to seriously limit physical activity or exercise, if you follow some modest requirements.
- Get a pre-exercise checkup from your doctor so that an exercise program can be tailored to you. Many people's bodies just won't do all the things they once did when they were, say, 25 years old. You are the best gauge of your limitations. But, whatever your limitations, there is still some kind of exercise you can do.
- Choose activities that help develop and maintain muscle strength and joint flexibility. An added benefit of these activities is they will help reduce the symptoms and discomfort of certain forms of arthritis.
- Do the activity or exercise at a low to moderate intensity to reduce the risk of injuries.
- Listen to your body. If your mobility is limited because of arthritis or aches and pains, cut down on your physical

activity, both the intensity and the length of time. Remember that age by itself is not a limitation. You can be physically active and gain the benefits of exercise at any age.

Exercise Can Be Categorized in Three Areas:

Aerobic exercise involves the heart, lungs, and muscles. This is the most beneficial type of exercise because it helps strengthen heart and blood vessels. It also burns calories and stored fat. It improves your overall physical fitness, too. Examples of aerobic exercise are walking, biking, swimming, and jogging.

Anaerobic exercise, such as weight training and resistance calisthenics, is high in intensity and uses energy stored in the muscles.

Anaerobic exercise increases muscle strength and has long-term benefits for the person with diabetes.

Flexibility exercise helps develop a good range of motion in the joints and muscles. This type of exercise includes stretching and bending, which are recommended as part of the warm-up and cool-down sessions before and after aerobic or anaerobic exercise.

Regular Exercise Options

If you choose to do regular exercise (as opposed to intense exercise), there are a wide variety of options. For indoor exercise (at home, in a shopping mall, at a community center, or a health club), you might choose:

- walking (on a track or through the hallways. Many malls have "mall walker" clubs.)
- aerobics
- stationary biking
- dancercize
- tennis
- racquetball or squash
- volleyball or handball
- swimming

For outdoor exercise, you might select:

- walking
- jogging

- hiking
- wall or mountain climbing
- biking
- swimming
- tennis, volleyball, handball
- softball
- golf
- roller or in-line skating

Intensive Exercise

Intensive exercise is not for everyone, especially those who are not in excellent physical shape or have diabetes complications. However, if you have followed a regular exercise program over the years, you may want to step up to the challenge of intensive exercise. Again, get your doctor's okay before you start such a program. You'll also need to increase the frequency of your blood glucose monitoring and make necessary adjustments to your management plan.

But, if you get the okay, here's an extra benefit you can expect from intensive exercise: Scientists have found that people who engage in intensive exercise live longer, have fewer heart attacks, and have lower cardiovascular death rates than people who engage in nonvigorous exercise.

A study conducted at Harvard University revealed that men who expended 2,500 calories a week on any activities lived significantly longer than men who burned fewer calories through exercise.

Vigorous, intensive exercise is defined as activities that raise the metabolic rate to six or more times the rate at rest. Such activities include brisk walking, jogging, singles tennis, lap-swimming, fast cycling, and doing heavy chores at home or in the yard.

To achieve the metabolic rate and burn 2,500 calories weekly, try one of the following:

- Walk at the rate of four to five miles per hour for 45 minutes, five times a week.
- Play one hour of singles tennis three days a week.
- Swim laps for three hours a week.

- Bike for one hour four times a week.
- Jog at six to seven miles an hour for three hours a week.
- In-line skate for two and a half hours a week.

Physical Activity Options

There are many options if you choose to add physical activity to your life, rather than formal exercise. Again, the benefits will be yours if you build three to four 10-minute sessions of physical activity into your daily routine. You can:

- Walk up the stairs at the shopping mall instead of taking an elevator.
- Park your car at the most distant part of the parking lot at the supermarket.
- Stash your remote controls for stereo and TV in a closet. Even a short walk to change channels or adjust the sound is good for you.
- Cancel home deliveries of newspapers and walk to the newsstand or newspaper dispenser each morning.
- Dust and vacuum the house two or three times a week. Remember the effectiveness of a hand-propelled broom or mop.
- Wash the kitchen and bathroom floors at least once a week. Wash the windows when they need it.
- Mow your lawn. Trade in your self-propelled lawnmower for a person-propelled one that mulches grass and helps the environment, too.
- Chop wood for your fireplace. Carry one or two pieces into the house at a time to avoid straining your back and to assure many trips.
- Carry small packages home from the store in your arms rather than in your car. Shop more often, but buy smaller quantities so you can carry these packages.
- Give away any electronic, time-saving devices. Use hand-driven devices like the ones your mother used: mixers, egg beaters, choppers, and grinders.

The following table shows how many calories you are likely to burn during various activities. The ranges correspond to how much you weigh. At 120 to 130 pounds, you'll burn the lower number of calories. At 190 or 200 pounds, you'll burn the higher number. Your weight range and the calories burned can be somewhere in between, so use this just to estimate.

Activity	Calories Burned in 30 minutes
AEROBIC DANCE	180 to 495
BICYCLING	
outdoors	120 to 690
indoors, stationary	150 to 690
BOWLING	90 to 180
CALISTHENICS	120 to 500
DANCING	90 to 500
GARDENING	90 to 360
GOLF (carry or pull bags)	90 to 360
JOGGING	
5 MPH	270 to 405
6 MPH	315 to 500
SKIING	
cross-country	180 to 690
downhill	120 to 400
SWIMMING	150 to 600
TENNIS	150 to 450
WALKING	
2 MPH	90 to 135
3 MPH	120 to 180
4 MPH	165 to 255

CHAPTER 8

Medications

Oral Hypoglycemic Agents

When diet and exercise don't seem to do the job in lowering blood glucose levels, many people with Type 2 diabetes can get help by taking a medication prescribed by their doctors. The medication is one of many in a class called oral hypoglycemic agents.

As the name states, these medications are taken orally. And they work to reduce blood glucose levels (*hypo*=low). These medications are not insulin, which must be taken by people with Type 1 diabetes and which may be taken by people with Type 2 diabetes, alone or along with an oral medication. Insulin can't be taken orally—it must be injected, or sometime in the future, may be taken as a nasal or mouth spray.

The first oral hypoglycemic agent was developed almost 60 years ago. It and its "cousins" have been widely and successfully used by millions of people with Type 2 diabetes throughout the world. This group of drugs has been called "first generation" oral agents, which must be taken two or three times a day in varying dosage strengths. Although there were a few side effects with the "first generation" agents, they were widely accepted and highly successful in lowering blood glucose levels for Type 2 diabetics—when these people also followed a "prescribed" meal and exercise plan.

It's important to remember that the drugs alone won't help control diabetes. They are only effective when they are used in combination with a meal and exercise plan.

In the mid- to late-1980s scientists developed a "second generation" family of oral hypoglycemic drugs that were sometimes more effective than the "first generation" and also carried with them the benefits of fewer side effects plus the convenience of one-a-day dosing.

As we close out the 20th century, we approach a period that is very exciting, for there are a number of new diabetes medications being developed and tested that offer even greater promise for the person with Type 2 diabetes. Some of these new medications may become available (by prescription) even before this book is printed.

Here is a brief summary of the available oral hypoglycemic agents, and a preview of what is on the horizon.

Sulfonylureas

These are the original oral hypoglycemic drugs that are available by prescription under the names: Orinase (tolbutamide), Dymelor (acetohexamide), Tolinase (tolazamide), and Diabinese (chlorpropamide). The dosages and duration of action of these drugs varies considerably.

The second generation sulfonylureas, which have fewer side effects, increased potency, and (usually) once a day dosage, are: Diabeta (glyburide), Micronase (glyburide), Glynase Prestab (micronized glyburide), Glucotrol (glipizide) and Glucotrol XL (glipizide), and Amaryl (glimepiride). The second generation agents were introduced in the late 1980s, except for Amaryl, which came on the market in 1996.

The sulfonylureas work by stimulating your pancreas to release more insulin and to improve the binding and intake of insulin in your muscle and fat cells. These drugs also reduce glucose production from your liver.

You need to take a sulfonylurea drug 30 minutes before you eat a meal (except for Glucotrol XL, which can be taken with a meal). Your doctor will probably start you on the lowest dose of the sulfonylurea and then gradually increase your dosage if your blood glucose levels increase. Although the second generation drugs generally are taken once a day, you may need two doses a day if you are at the maximum strength level.

If you have an allergy to sulfa drugs, you may be allergic to this class of drugs. You may not react favorably to these drugs if your blood glucose levels are extremely elevated due to stress, infection, surgery, liver, or kidney disease. You should not take these drugs if you are pregnant. You will not benefit from these drugs if you have Type 1 diabetes (where you require insulin injections).

Biguanides

Only one of this class of drugs is currently available in the United States: Glucophage (metformin). This agent is prescribed for use by people with Type 2 diabetes alone (along with diet and exercise) or in combination with other oral agents (sulfonylureas) or with insulin injections.

Metformin works by increasing the uptake of glucose and utilization of glucose by muscle cells and by improving insulin sensitivity. It also decreases production of glucose by the liver, and decreases absorption of glucose in the intestine.

When used alone, metformin does not cause low blood glucose reactions or hyperinsulinemia. In addition, this drug may help you lose weight and may lower your blood fat levels.

Starting dosage usually is one 500 mg tablet, twice a day. In some people a single 850 mg tablet once a day can be effective. Dosage can be increased up to a total of 2,500 mg a day, after which time your doctor may add a sulfonylurea drug to your mix.

This type of medication may have a serious side effect which is called lactic acidosis. Your doctor will want to check on this during regular visits or if you report symptoms that include weakness, fatigue, unusual muscle pain, difficulty in breathing, a sudden or unusual stomach discomfort, lightheadedness, or change in your heartbeat.

If you have liver or kidney problems, or are pregnant, you should not take this drug. It is generally stopped if you have to be in the hospital.

Alpha-Glucosidase Inhibitors

The two drugs on the market at this time are Precose (acarbose) and Glyset Tablets (miglitol), which can be used alone (along with diet and exercise) or in combination with a sulfonylurea.

These drugs slow the absorption of complex carbohydrates in the foods you eat during the digestive process in your intestines. This, in effect, lowers the increase of blood glucose levels you will experience following the eating of a meal.

You need to take these agents with the first bite of food you eat at mealtimes. You'll be started on a low dose, which will be increased gradually over the next few months.

Most of the side effects (flatulence and loose or frequent stools) occur at the beginning of treatment and will disappear as dosage is increased.

You should not take these drugs if you are pregnant or if you have kidney problems or certain kinds of intestinal disease. They should not be used if you are taking Amylase or Pancreatin or have gastrointestinal side effects with other medications.

Thiazolidinediones

One of the newer drugs available to people with Type 2 diabetes is called Rezulin (troglitazone). This drug belongs to a new class of drugs known as insulin sensitivity enhancers.

This drug increases insulin sensitivity in the liver, and muscle and fat tissue, thereby making the insulin you produce (or inject) more effective in lowering blood glucose levels.

Although initially indicated for use by people with Type 2 diabetes who are injecting insulin (and are having difficulty in controlling blood glucose levels), this drug may be prescribed for you, particularly if other oral agents have not proved effective.

This agent can be taken with a meal, once a day, with the dosage determined by the results of frequent blood glucose monitoring. The drug should not be used if you have hepatic disease, congestive heart failure, or if you are pregnant. It is not yet approved for use by children, and is not to be used by anyone with Type 1 diabetes.

Recent reports of serious side effects resulting from use of this drug are currently (1998) being evaluated in clinical studies. Check with your doctor regarding any concerns you may have. The U.S. Food and Drug Administration and the manufacturer say that the benefits of this drug outweigh any risks, but monthly liver function tests are recommended if you are taking this drug.

Another drug in this class of insulin sensitivity enhancers is Avandia (rosiglitazone maleate), which is in advanced clinical trials and has shown promise in lowering blood glucose levels with few if any side effects.

Meglitinides

The first drug to be marketed in this new class of oral agents is Prandin (repaglinide), which quickly increases insulin secretion when food is eaten. It is taken 15 to 30 minutes before a meal, two to four times a day. Prandin may be taken alone or in combination with metformin.

On the Horizon

There are a number of new drugs that are now in clinical trials that may be marketed by the time you read this book (or shortly thereafter). Here is a capsule summary of some of those being developed.

Ergoset, a low-dose, fast-release oral formulation of bromocriptine (a drug currently used to treat Parkinson's disease), has been shown in clinical trials to be at least as good as existing oral hypoglycemic drugs, with a low risk of side effects.

Targretin, a drug tested against various cancers, has been found to intervene directly between insulin and the protein inside cells to regulate blood glucose. This is a new approach to diabetes treatment, which also holds promise as an agent to delay or prevent the onset of diabetes.

Another class of drugs is being studied in the hopes of finding an agent that has the potential of destroying molecules that attack the pancreas, cause resistance to insulin and may contribute to the development of serious complications of diabetes.

In other research studies that may produce marketable medication further in the future is a powdered insulin that can be

Oral Hypoglycemic Agents Presently Available in the U.S. and Canada

Drug Name	Trade Name	Dosage	Duration	Special Properties
Tolbutamide	Orinase	500 mg starting dose; maximum 2 to 3 grams daily. Taken 2 to 3 times a day.	6 to 10 hours	Shortest-acting sulfonylurea, with lowest frequency of side effects.
Acetohexamide	Dymelor	250 mg starting dose; maximum 1 to 1 1/2 grams daily. Taken twice a day.	12 to 18 hours	User must have normal liver and kidney functions.
Tolazamide	Tolinase	100 mg starting dose; maximum 1 gram daily. Taken 1 to 2 times a day.	18 to 24 hours	Peak action 3 to 4 hours after ingestion; extended duration of action.
Chlorpropamide	Diabinese	100 to 250 mg starting dose; maximum 500 mg daily. Taken once a day.	More than 24 hours	Longest-acting oral agent; side effects include alcohol facial flush effect and lowering of sodium levels.
Glimepiride	Amaryl	1 to 4 mg, maximum 8 mg, once a day	24 hours	Newer agent

Drug Name	Trade Name	Dosage	Duration	Special Properties
Glipizide	Glucotrol	2.5 to 5 mg starting dose; maximum 40 mg daily. Taken 1 to 2 times.	16 to 24 hours	Second-generation agent that is 100 to 150 times more potent than tolbutamide.
Glyburide	Micronase, Diabeta, Glynase	1.5 to 5 mg starting dose; maximum 20 mg daily. Taken 1 to 2 times a day.	12 to 24 hours	Second-generation agent. User should have normal kidney function.
Metformin	Glucophage	500 mg starting dose; maximum 2500 mg daily. Taken twice a day.	6 to 12 hours	Buildup of lactic acid possible so not advised for people with liver or kidney problems.
Acarbose	Precose	25 mg three times a day; max 100tid		Take dose with first bite of each meal.
Miglitol	Glyset	25 mg three times daily; max 100tid		Take dose before meals.
Troglitazone	Rezulin	200 mg once daily; max 600 mg		Enhances efficacy of insulin injections. Toxicity warrants frequent liver function tests.
Repaglinide	Prandin	0.5 to 2 mg starting dose; max 16 mg daily; Taken before each meal.		Enhances insulin secretion.

inhaled rather than injected, and a compound based on a tropical plant that has been used by native cultures to treat symptoms of diabetes. Also, HOE (an experimental, long-acting insulin analog) is hoped to best mimic the normal basal secretion of insulin when it is available.

Insulin

Insulin is a hormone secreted by the beta cells in your pancreas gland. It controls the rate glucose (or sugar) is taken up by cells in the body. Once glucose is within the cells, it is burned as fuel to keep all body functions running. If glucose does not get into the cells, it piles up in the bloodstream. When this happens, blood glucose levels soar and the risks of diabetes complications increase dramatically.

When your body does not produce enough insulin, or cannot effectively use the insulin it produces (a condition called insulin resistance), something must be done to solve this problem. For some people, losing weight by following an eating plan and starting an exercise program is enough. For others, the eating plan and the exercise program may be combined with medication, such as the oral hypoglycemic agents shown earlier in the table in this chapter.

If these two approaches fail, however, insulin injections are required to keep blood glucose levels within the normal range. Many people with Type 2 diabetes do need insulin injections. All people with Type 1 diabetes depend on insulin injections. (People with Type 1 diabetes do not produce any insulin, so they need daily insulin injections to live.)

Currently, insulin must be injected to be effective. Since insulin is a protein, it would be destroyed by your body if you took it orally. Although scientists are working on ways to make insulin effective as a nasal spray or in capsule form, these experimental methods have not yet proven to be practical. Aerosolized insulin that is inhaled through the mouth, similar to the inhalers for asthma, is also being tested and appears to be less irritating than the nasal spray.

If you require insulin injections, you should keep in mind that insulin (like oral agents, or even an eating plan) does not control diabetes by itself. In fact, if you inject insulin and don't eat enough food, or if you exercise too much, you could experience a serious low blood glucose attack (hypoglycemia). If you eat too much, or if you don't exercise, and you still inject insulin, you will probably experience high blood glucose levels and eventually an unwanted increase in your weight.

Like everything else in your diabetes management plan, it's important to balance each element to achieve success. In the past, doctors usually prescribed a single injection of insulin each day. Today most doctors recommend multiple injections. Some people require two or three injections daily for best results. Your doctor will develop an insulin injection schedule that fits your lifestyle and that best helps control your diabetes.

There are different sources of insulin. Pork and beef were once the primary types of insulin. Today most insulin is genetically engineered and synthesized. It is called "human" insulin because it is identical to the insulin our bodies produce.

There are different types of insulin, which vary in how quickly they start to work (their onset of action), their peak of action, and the duration of their action (see the following chart).

Action of Available Insulins

Family	Type	Onset (hours)	Peak (hours)	Duration (hours)
NPH	Regular	1–2	3–4	6
	NPH	4	8–12	18
	PZI	4	18–24	36
Lente	Semilente	1–2	3–4	6
	Lente	4	8–12	18–24
	Ultralente	4	None (if given properly)	18
Insulin analogs	Lispro	1/4	1–2	3

Finally, there are different strengths of insulin and different manufacturers. The most commonly used insulin concentration in the U.S. is U-100, which means 100 units of insulin per milliliter. Outside the U.S., the most commonly used concentration is U-40, or 40 units of insulin per milliliter.

If you are just starting insulin injections, be sure your diabetes health care professional teaches you how and where to inject insulin. You'll learn how to store insulin, how to draw insulin from its vials, and how to rotate injection sites.

Please note: You should never change the brand, dosage, or strength of insulin without instructions from your diabetes health care professional.

The most common way to inject insulin is with a needle and syringe. Most needles and syringes are packaged as one-use disposables. Fortunately, needles are made sharper and thinner than ever before. They can pierce the skin almost painlessly. Such products are inexpensive and very convenient, but you need to be careful about disposing needles so others won't be punctured.

Note that it is illegal to put used needles in everyday trash. Ask your trash hauler for a special container for sharp medical products and the phone number to call for pickup and replacement containers when the container is full.

To save money, you may be tempted to reuse a disposable needle and syringe. This may be okay under certain circumstances, particularly if you learn how to keep the needle free of contamination and you protect the sharp point.

Syringe sizes correspond with the concentration of the insulin. Make extra sure you use U-100 syringes with U-100 insulin.

When you inject insulin you must puncture the skin and inject the insulin into fatty tissue, such as in the upper arm, top and outsides of the thigh, buttocks, or abdomen. Insulin is absorbed most rapidly and evenly when injected into the fatty tissue in the abdomen. Arms and thighs are second-choice sites, followed by the buttocks. To avoid injection-caused problems, such as lipoatrophy and hypertrophy, rotate your injection sites and avoid using the same spot day after day.

In addition to the needle/syringe injection method, there are some alternative insulin delivery systems. While these are considerably more expensive than using a needle and syringe, they are very helpful to people who cannot take insulin injections.

INSULIN PEN: A compact, pen-like device containing a cartridge filled with a specific amount of insulin, or a combination of two types of insulin. You change the needle, usually for each injection, and set the dosage by rotating the head of the pen or counting the number of times the plunger is pressed. Newer pens are disposable after the insulin in the cartridge is used up (up to 150 units). Premixed insulin cartridges (in 70/30 ratios) are now available.

SPRAY INJECTOR: A device that uses air pressure to blow a stream of insulin through the pores of your skin. You draw insulin up from the standard vial, set the specific dosage by rotating a section of this device, then place the head of the device on your skin. Activate the spray. This is an ideal choice for those with "needle phobia."

AUTOMATIC INJECTOR: This device uses a spring mechanism to depress the syringe plunger and insert the needle through your skin. You place the needle and syringe (loaded with the correct amount of insulin) into the device and press a button that releases the spring mechanism. This option is also good for people who don't care for needles or anyone with physical restrictions that interfere with the regular injection technique.

INSULIN PUMP: This automated device releases insulin from a reservoir through tubing and a needle inserted in the skin on a 24-hour basis. The insulin pump frequently is used by people with Type 1, insulin-dependent diabetes who have difficulty maintaining blood glucose control with the standard needle and syringe. Implantable pumps have also been used successfully in Type 2 patients in research settings.

ASSISTIVE DEVICES: If you have sight or dexterity problems, there are devices available to assist with insulin injections. These include aids that help people read the numbers and lines on a syringe (known as a syringe magnifier), and others that hold a syringe and insulin vial to make loading easier or that pinch your skin to leave your hand free to handle the syringe.

When you first start injecting insulin, you will have to change your blood glucose monitoring schedule, increasing the frequency and changing the times of monitoring. Instead of checking your blood glucose after a meal (which is recommended for Type 2 diabetes controlled by diet and exercise or by diet, exercise, and an oral agent), you will be advised to measure your blood glucose before you eat.

This pre-meal blood glucose information will enable you to adjust your insulin dosage and/or food at that meal so that the action of the insulin matches the food intake. Sound complicated? Don't worry, with proper instructions from your diabetes health care professional, you'll soon find that this sort of fine-tuning becomes routine.

Just how often and when you monitor depends on how many injections you take each day, how closely you follow your eating plan and exercise program, and how your blood glucose control responds.

Another important consideration is the proper care of insulin. Here are the rules:

- Store insulin vials currently being used at room temperature.
- Store extra vials of insulin in a cool place, but not the refrigerator or freezer.
- Protect insulin from extreme cold or extreme heat.
- Do not use a vial of insulin beyond the expiration date printed on the label.
- Store pre-filled insulin syringes in the refrigerator, but not for more than 14 days.
- Take extra precautions when you travel. Pack extra insulin in an insulated case (not in your luggage or the glove compartment or trunk of your car).

Other Medications

If you are like most adults, you are probably taking prescription or nonprescription medications for health problems other than diabetes. It could be as simple as an aspirin for a headache or cough medicine. Perhaps you take a nonsteroidal anti-inflammatory drug (NSAID) when your arthritis flares up. Anti-hypertensive drugs to control high blood pressure are also common.

Most of these medications are relatively safe to use, but they may all have some effect on your diabetes control. Because of this potential, you should be especially careful about taking any medications. For instance, anti-fungal medicines can lower the effect of oral agents.

First, be sure to inform your diabetes doctor about any drugs you use that have been prescribed by another doctor. Be sure to tell the doctor also about any nonprescription drugs you use to treat minor ailments. This information will be recorded on your medical history and checked before the doctor considers adding a diabetes medication to your management plan.

Also, check with your pharmacist when you fill a new prescription and before you get a nonprescription medication from the drugstore shelf. The pharmacist can check to see if there are interactions between your new prescriptions and other medications you are taking. If there are interactions, your pharmacist should contact your doctor before filling the prescription. The doctor and pharmacist can then recommend an alternative.

Pharmacists can also advise people on how to select nonprescription remedies that don't interfere with diabetes management programs. Among other things, you'll want to avoid nonprescription drugs that contain hidden sugars or alcohol that can upset blood glucose control.

You'll want to check with your diabetes health care team before buying and using any nonprescription remedies for foot, eye, or skin problems. Some products can do more harm than good.

Here is some information about the four most common types of medication used by adults, with or without diabetes:

Hypertension Medications

Millions of adults have high blood pressure (hypertension). As someone with Type 2 diabetes, you are at increased risk for hypertension. If you are overweight and over the age of 40, you are at even higher risk for hypertension. Unless hypertension is effectively controlled, it can lead to stroke and death.

Like many of the symptoms of Type 2 diabetes, symptoms of hypertension are not easily detected. Usually a blood pressure measurement is the only way to determine if blood pressure is above normal. Then, once you take steps to control hypertension, you won't be able to feel when your blood pressure drops to normal. Both these facts present problems: first with diagnosis, secondly with control.

Fortunately, you probably see your doctor for checkups regularly. During these checkups your blood pressure will be measured. If you are diagnosed as having hypertension, your doctor will prescribe a management plan similar to this:

- Eat a well balanced diet (If you are salt-sensitive, your doctor will recommend that you cut down on adding salt to your foods and avoid eating salty snacks.)
- Eliminate excess weight
- Exercise regularly
- Cope with stress effectively
- Eliminate alcohol and tobacco products

Sound familiar? It should because it's the same advice given to people diagnosed with Type 2 diabetes.

If these recommendations don't do the job of lowering blood pressure, doctors often prescribe a hypertension medication. Despite the name, hypertension medications do not "cure" hypertension. It is a lifelong condition, so once you start medication, you'll have to stay on it. Some people remain on the original prescription, some move to a combination of drugs, and others are prescribed more powerful drugs.

Because a blood pressure check is the only way to tell if it is normal or abnormal, willpower and intelligence play a big part in sticking with a blood pressure treatment plan. Fortunately, many prescription medications are available to control hypertension. When taken as prescribed, they not only lower blood pressure, but they also may affect blood glucose levels—either up or down.

Some medications cause fatigue, which can make you want to skip exercise and physical activities. If you skip exercise, blood glucose levels will rise. To overcome this desire for inactivity, you will have to use a lot of self-motivation.

Some medicine can also damage the kidneys or eyes. If you notice any persistent side effects, contact your doctor immediately. An alternate drug or a dosage change may clear up the problem.

Almost all hypertension medications have the potential to reduce blood pressure too low. This can result in dizziness, especially if you stand up quickly or when you get out of bed in the morning. Be aware of this problem so you can take precautions to avoid falls. If dizziness persists, contact your doctor for advice.

There are a few more cautions to remember:

• Don't self-treat hypertension with home remedies. These don't work and may only increase the risks for stroke.
• Don't take a hypertension medication (or ANY prescription medication) that has been prescribed for a family member or friend. Although this person may have hypertension like you, the medication that he or she takes may have adverse effects on you and your diabetes.

When you first start taking a hypertension medication, you should monitor your blood glucose more frequently to see how the medication affects blood glucose levels. Check right before you take the medication and one hour after. Then record the measurement in a diary or log. Let your doctor know if there's a major change in blood glucose levels after you have been taking the medication for a long period.

As you know, prescription medications work in different ways. Among the most popular are ACE inhibitors (angiotensin converting enzyme inhibitors). These drugs are particularly effective in people with Type 2 diabetes since they cause few side effects and don't damage the kidneys.

Another class of drugs are called alpha or beta blockers. Alpha blockers are more commonly prescribed for people with diabetes because they don't have a major effect on blood glucose levels. Beta blockers are widely used for people with heart problems. They not only lower blood pressure, they also lower blood glucose levels. Use caution and be prepared to detect and treat potential low blood glucose attacks if this drug is prescribed for you.

Cholesterol and Triglyceride Medications

It's a good bet that everyone has heard the risks associated with having too much cholesterol, triglycerides, and fats, in general.

The media messages are true. Americans, especially, eat too many fatty and high-cholesterol foods, which greatly increases our risk for heart disease and strokes.

We've been told to eat low-fat and low-cholesterol foods. We've been told to add fish oil, olive oil, and canola oil to our diets and to get rid of butter. We've been told to increase our good cholesterol and to reduce our bad cholesterol. It's been almost too much. But there's a lot of truth in the advice.

People with diabetes are at increased risk for heart disease and cardiovascular problems, including stroke. The risk for heart disease grows for people with diabetes if they are over 40 and carrying around extra body weight.

Unfortunately, many people have been eating a high-fat diet most of their lives. They probably haven't done much in the way of regular exercise over the years either. Their lifestyle, eating and exercise habits, and genes have led to the diagnosis of Type 2 diabetes. Along with high blood glucose levels, they probably also have high cholesterol and triglyceride levels.

What's a person to do? If you are facing these types of challenges, the answer is quite simple. Follow your diabetes management program to the absolute best of your ability. What has been prescribed for diabetes control also is the answer for cholesterol and triglyceride control. Your eating plan is designed to lower your fat and calorie intake. The same eating plan is recommended to control cholesterol and triglyceride levels.

Your exercise program is designed to tune up your body, to increase your cardiovascular fitness, and to burn off excess calories. That same exercise program also works to help lower cholesterol and triglyceride levels.

You've been advised to learn how to cope with stress, to stop smoking, and to be moderate in your alcohol intake. That same advice is given to people at risk for heart disease.

When diet and exercise alone don't work, a variety of prescription medications are available. These medications, however, won't work unless you follow the prescribed eating and exercise plans.

Some medications work to lower cholesterol. Others lower triglycerides. Your doctor may prescribe a two-medication approach if your problem involves both cholesterol and triglycerides.

Arthritis and Pain Medications

Millions of adults suffer from osteoarthritis or rheumatoid arthritis. Most take one or more medications to treat the pain, stiffness, and swelling that arthritis produces. These same symptoms are some of the most common problems of aging. Unfortunately, people with diabetes are at increased risk for these problems if they don't keep blood glucose levels under good control.

We can't stop the aging process or cure arthritis, but we can help by maintaining good glucose control and taking care of our physical and emotional selves. Still, most everyone will occasionally feel pain and swelling in the joints of their fingers or feet, in their elbows or shoulders, or in their neck and back.

When these pains flare up, many people turn to aspirin, Tylenol, or a nonsteroid anti-inflammatory drug (NSAID), such as Naprosyn or ibuprofen, which are available without prescription. Or perhaps their doctor has prescribed one of the more potent NSAIDs with powerful pain-killing action.

All of these medications have the potential to upset your blood glucose control. That's why you should check your blood glucose before you start a new medication and one hour after to see any effects the medication has.

Your pharmacist can advise you on safe and effective nonprescription choices, and your doctor can prescribe medications that are effective but have little effect on blood glucose control and are relatively free of side effects. Remember that the more potent the pain-killing medication, the greater its potential for producing undesirable side effects. With NSAIDs, the major side effects are stomach and gastrointestinal distress and bleeding (sometimes leading to ulcers). Many people with Type 2 diabetes are encouraged to take a baby aspirin a day to lower cardiovascular risk. Ask your doctor if this is appropriate for you.

Cough and Cold Medications

There is no cure for the common cold—at least not yet. There are lots of medications that work, however, to relieve the symptoms of a cold: coughing, sneezing, stuffy nose, you know the rest.

But these cough and cold remedies may also contain ingredients that can upset blood glucose control and raise blood pressure. Some contain alcohol. Some contain sugar, often hidden under unfamiliar ingredient names.

Talk to your pharmacist before you buy a cough or cold remedy. The pharmacist can tell you which brands will relieve your symptoms without disrupting blood glucose control and raising blood pressure. If a pharmacist is not available, try a single-symptom medication (such as medicine for a cough or medicine for a stuffy nose) rather than a multiple symptom "shotgun" medication. You'll not only save money, you'll lower your risks of unwanted side effects.

CHAPTER 9

Monitoring Your Health

How Are You Doing?

That's a question friends ask as a greeting, but it's also a question you should ask yourself every day. You can find out just how well you are doing by monitoring certain things—sort of like checking the oil in your car before a long trip. If the dipstick shows you have enough oil, then you can start the engine and begin your trip. If the oil is low, you make adjustments—in this case, adding oil to the correct level.

The same holds true for your personal checkups as you check the functions of your body and status of certain "components." If everything is okay, then you have the go-ahead to proceed with your daily activities. If something isn't quite right, then you need to make adjustments.

Time and energy spent checking a car and correcting problems helps avoid costly repairs in the future. Time and energy you spend self-monitoring and making the right adjustments can prevent major, costly health problems in the future.

Remember, though, checking your oil without correcting the problem won't save the engine. In the same way, just checking your blood glucose, weight, or blood pressure won't improve your health unless you make changes that will solve problems and improve your health.

Blood Glucose Monitoring

Perhaps the most important thing you can do is to check your blood glucose levels. When you know where your blood glucose levels are, you can then fine-tune your diabetes control. You can adjust the amount and kind of food you eat, you can adjust the amount of exercise you do, and you can even change the dosage of medicine you may be taking to control blood glucose levels. That may seem like work, but the work is worthwhile if you can "normalize" your blood glucose levels. When this happens, you will not only look and feel better, you'll also be reducing your risks for complications.

Today, we can thank modern science for developing easy-to-use and relatively inexpensive blood glucose measurement tools: palm-sized electronic glucose meters, no-fuss glucose strips, and almost-painless finger sticking devices. These aids were not available to the generation of people with diabetes who preceded you. If you have had diabetes for more than 20 years, you know that the only measurement method available when you were first diagnosed was the urine sugar test (and this test could only indicate when sugar levels were high, not when they were low).

Progress in manufacturing has enabled new glucose measuring equipment to be simpler to use, more reliable, smaller, and even less expensive. On the distant horizon are glucose measuring tools that won't require you to stick your finger to obtain a drop of blood to be analyzed. Scientists are working on an implantable sensor that will display blood glucose levels on a wristwatch-style receiver. Development efforts are underway, but for the time being, you still have to depend on current technology.

Why Monitor Blood Glucose?

You may ask why you need to monitor your blood glucose. The major reason is to find out if your blood glucose level is above or below normal at the time of the measurement. If your blood glucose level is a little bit above or below the range that you and your physician have established as "normal" for you, then you can review what you have or haven't been doing that may have sent the reading up or down. For example, it may be that you couldn't

A TOUCH OF DIABETES

exercise; possibly you ate a second helping at lunch or skipped a meal entirely. Here's the good news: A single, slightly high or low measurement is nothing to get upset about. If you can identify why the reading is high or low, that's excellent. You can try tomorrow to avoid repeating what you did or did not do today.

However, a number of slightly high or low measurements (at the same time of day for several days in a row) is something that you should be concerned about. That repetition of "highs" or "lows" shows a potentially harmful pattern that needs to be changed before major damage is done in your body.

As you may know, blood glucose test results in the United States are expressed in milligrams per deciliter (mg/dL). Outside the U.S., blood glucose is often measured in millimols per liter (mmol/L). To convert a test result in mg/dL into mmol/L, simply divide the number by 18 for its approximate equivalent.

You can use a diabetes diary (or any other kind of log book) to record all of your blood glucose measurements (along with other pertinent information). Check the diary every few days to determine if there is a pattern of above-normal measurements. If you see a pattern that is not quite right, contact your diabetes health care professional to find out what you need to do to bring your blood glucose levels back into the normal range. Many models will also give an average blood glucose reading. This information is helpful as you learn skills to lower your average.

While you are looking for patterns of blood glucose control, be wary of a single extremely high or low blood glucose reading. This should be considered a red flag that requires action.

Hopefully, before you experience any blood glucose control problems, you will have talked with your diabetes health care professional about what you should do when you get a "red-flag" reading. That way you'll be armed with options and know what to do. If you still have questions, though, call your doctor or diabetes health professional for advice.

Another major reason to monitor blood glucose levels and keep them in good control is that you lower your risks for diabetes complications and life-threatening problems such as heart attacks and strokes. These potential problems should not be ignored.

What is the Normal Range for Blood Glucose?

Time of Measurement	Ideal	Acceptable
Fasting, or before a meal	70–110 mg/dL (3.9–6.1 mmol/L)	60–126 mg/dL (3.3–7 mmol/L)
One hour after a meal	90–150 mg/dL (5–8.3 mmol/L)	80–160 mg/dL (4.4–8.9 mmol/L)
Two hours after a meal	80–120 mg/dL (4.4–6.7 mmol/L)	70–120 mg/dL (3.9–6.7 mmol/L)
Three hours after a meal	80–110 mg/dL (4.4–6.1 mmol/L)	70–120 mg/dL (3.9–6.7 mmol/L)

Young children and elderly persons can maintain blood glucose levels on the high side of their established range. Pregnant women should aim for blood glucose levels that average between 90 and 100 mg/dL (4.4 and 5.5 mmol/L).

From Morton's Journal

For me, blood glucose monitoring is the simplest task in my diabetes self-management program. It's really a no-brainer to operate one of the newer meters. It's a fool-proof operation, and it really is painless when I use one of the finger-sticking devices. In 30 seconds I get a reading, and that reading tells me just how good (or bad) I have been.

Sure, sometimes I go off my healthy meal plan and eat a larger than "prescribed" portion of a rich (but tasty) food. And I have been known to have a martini before dinner. The meter, however, is my conscience. It tells all, and then I have to deal with the results. The meter (or the results I get from it) helps me to better know my body and how that body reacts to food, exercise, and the stresses of life. I think it is a good thing.

Sometimes I get a reading that is way off the scale—either too high or too low. When this happens, I just do another test. The second reading usually is within the range that I expect. I guess that sometimes my technique is off and I use too little or too much blood. Or, maybe the computer inside the meter is having a bad day (just like the one on which I am writing this journal).

Perhaps my attitude toward meters is affected by my past. When the first meter was introduced in the late 1960s, it was a clunker that required constant calibration. To stick your finger you used the tip of a scalpel. A large drop of blood had to be placed on the reagent pad on a strip, and then it had to be blotted (correctly) within a set time. Too much or too little time, too little or too much blotting, and the results were way off. The meter needed to be cleaned regularly or you'd get skewed results. To top things off, the meter had to be plugged into an electric socket, and the strips had to be kept in airtight containers. One slip and you were a goner.

Thanks to people with diabetes who liked to self monitor, and to the health professionals who supported the idea that diabetics could assume responsibility for self-management of their disease, the meters and the self-monitoring process has been streamlined to its current simplified level. And I can hardly wait to see what is coming next.

It's true that you may never develop complications or have a heart attack. On the other hand, it's also true that you may be in great danger of these if you don't keep your blood glucose levels in good control. The stakes are too high to gamble with your life and health.

Here are some facts for consideration. If blood glucose levels stay above normal for long periods, complications can occur, including:

- Retinopathy, or eye damage, that can lead to partial or complete blindness.
- Neuropathy, or nerve damage, that produces loss of sensation and/or pain in the legs or hands. It can also affect the ability to digest food.

- Nephropathy, or kidney function damage, that can lead to kidney failure and death.
- Problems with large blood vessels that can lead to heart attacks and strokes.
- Sexual function problems that can lead to impotence in men and vaginal dryness in women.

It can take years for these health problems to develop. Fortunately, you can take action to prevent them.

There's good scientific evidence that tight control of blood glucose levels can prevent complications or make them less severe. Tight control may also reverse some damage if the damage is not permanent. The evidence was produced in the nationwide Diabetes Control and Complications Trial (DCCT), which ended in 1993. The study found that in people under tight control:

- Eye damage decreased by 76 percent
- Kidney damage decreased by 35 to 56 percent
- Nerve damage decreased by 60 percent

While the DCCT studied people with Type 1 diabetes, an even newer study has shown that tight control of blood glucose levels significantly reduces the chances of eye and kidney damage in people with Type 2 diabetes.

The United Kingdom Prospective Diabetes Study (UKPDS) studied over 5,000 people with Type 2 diabetes, some for 20 years. In the study, tight control reduced (by 25 percent) the chances of developing eye and kidney damage. Lowering blood glucose levels (as measured by a hemoglobin A1c test, which is discussed on page 103) also resulted in a 35 percent reduction in damage to the eyes, kidneys, and nerves, and a 25 percent reduction in diabetes-related deaths.

How and When to Monitor Blood Glucose

How to monitor has become relatively easy, thanks to technology. Manufacturers of blood glucose monitoring equipment have worked hard to make the procedure relatively simple and foolproof.

The procedure is simple, but it still must be done in the right order to get accurate results. And inaccurate readings of blood glucose levels are not only a waste of time, energy, and money, but can also be dangerous.

Currently, for all home blood-glucose monitoring systems, you need to prick a fingertip with a lancing device (either built-in or separate) to obtain a drop of blood. Then you place this drop on a chemically-treated pad on a strip or stick. Most systems then require you to place this strip in a receptacle in the glucose meter. However, with some systems, you place the strip into the meter first, then apply the blood.

The electronics in the meter then time the reaction between the blood and chemically-treated strip or stick, translate the results into numbers, which are displayed on a screen, and, in some systems, store the results in memory. For most systems, results are ready within 60 seconds, although there's one more important step: you need to record the results in a diary or log—even if the meter has its own memory.

Some of the more sophisticated meters have computer modems that allow you to transmit your blood glucose measurements directly to your computer or one in the office of your diabetes health care professional for analysis. Your health care professional can teach you about the different blood glucose measurement systems and train you on how to properly use the system you choose.

Keep in mind that many health insurance plans (including Medicare) will reimburse you for the purchase of a meter when a doctor prescribes it, in writing, as part of a diabetes treatment plan. Some health insurance plans also provide reimbursement for the purchase of glucose test strips.

So, are you wondering how often you should monitor your blood glucose? The answer is straightforward: "As often as possible."

By knowing your blood glucose level, you are free to do exactly what you want to do with your life. That's just one of the benefits of frequent blood glucose monitoring.

But don't go overboard. There's no need to measure your blood glucose every hour. But you should establish a monitoring schedule that you'll be comfortable with and one that you'll be likely to follow.

When you first start to monitor your blood glucose, you should do it a few times each day until the procedure becomes a normal part of your lifestyle. This frequent monitoring schedule is also necessary if you have recently been diagnosed as having Type 2 diabetes.

Here's a basic monitoring schedule effective for most people with Type 2 diabetes. Remember, however, that you and your doctor will set a schedule specifically for you, so these guidelines are general.

DIABETES CONTROL WITH DIET AND EXERCISE ALONE: Self-monitor before breakfast and one hour after each meal, every other day or three times a week or if you eat a new food or feel "funny."

DIABETES CONTROL WITH DIET, EXERCISE, AND AN ORAL HYPOGLYCEMIC AGENT: Self-monitor before breakfast and one hour after each meal every other day.

DIABETES CONTROL WITH DIET, EXERCISE, AND MULTIPLE INSULIN INJECTIONS: Self-monitor before each meal, plus one hour after each meal every day.

Again, your blood glucose monitoring schedule should be tailored to you and your diabetes. If you control your diabetes with diet and exercise alone, you may have to monitor your blood glucose after each meal and at bedtime a few times a week. If you add an oral agent to the mix, you may want to monitor your blood glucose daily. If you use insulin, you'll probably need to test before you inject and after a meal, so you can adjust either your food intake or insulin dosage to ensure your insulin and eating plan are matched.

In addition to regularly scheduled measurements, you should monitor your blood glucose when you don't feel quite right. It may be the heat and humidity, or it may be high blood glucose that makes you feel like a wet dishcloth. Talk with your diabetes health care professional about setting a blood glucose monitoring schedule for normal days and one when you have a minor illness, are under great stress, or are experiencing poor control.

If you're planning strenuous exercise, it's a good idea to check your blood glucose before you start. Here are some guidelines:

- Wait before you exercise if your readings are far above normal. You'll need to make adjustments in your pre-exercise meal or medication dosage and timing to bring blood glucose levels into a more normal range before exercising. Check with your doctor to set your exercise glucose "limits."
- Eat something if the pre-exercise reading is below normal. Don't risk an exercise-induced low blood glucose attack.
- Be prepared for emergencies (such as low blood glucose during or after exercise) by carrying a quick-sugar source or snack. Also, make sure your exercise partner knows what to do if you show signs of low blood glucose.

Frequent monitoring is also helpful when you are under stress because blood glucose levels may soar. Typical stress-inducers include any kind of major change in your life (i.e., getting married, moving to a new house, changing jobs, death of a loved one). If your self-measurement confirms the effects of stress, then you should make the appropriate adjustments in your management program and implement stress-reducing techniques such as relaxation, meditation, or yoga.

Blood glucose monitoring can also help people lose excess weight. Here's how:

Certain foods have hidden calories with glucose-raising effects. Learn how specific foods affect blood glucose levels. Hidden calories not only can send blood glucose levels soaring, they can also contribute to fat stores.

Measure your blood glucose before you eat a regular-sized portion of a particular food and then one hour after. Avoid those foods that send blood glucose levels soaring; choose foods that have a moderate effect. This will help your weight-loss efforts.

See how blood glucose levels on average for a week go down

when you lose just a few pounds. A ten-pound weight loss has a dramatic effect on blood glucose levels. This tangible result is great motivation during weight-loss programs.

What Glucose Monitoring Won't Do

Blood glucose monitoring does little if anything by itself. Monitoring alone won't reduce weight, prevent complications, or bring glucose levels within normal range. Blood glucose monitoring provides information, nothing more.

To get benefits from blood glucose monitoring, you need to act on the information that you obtain. First you need to learn from a diabetes health care professional what you can and should do when blood glucose levels are outside the normal range:

- You may need to adjust your eating plan.
- You may need to adjust your exercise or physical activity schedule.
- You may need to adjust the timing and/or dosage of your diabetes medication.
- Or you may need to change medication or start taking insulin injections.

With guidance, you'll learn how to fine-tune your diabetes management program and balance your food, exercise, and medication. Blood glucose monitoring provides the tool to achieve this balance.

Other Diabetes Tests

In the past, people with diabetes checked their control by using urine sugar tests, either tablets or strips. During the past decade or so, most people with diabetes have switched from urine tests to blood glucose monitoring. If you are still using a urine sugar test, it's time to discuss a change with your doctor or diabetes health care professional.

The only urine test you may be asked to do in a modern diabetes management programs is a urine ketone test. As a person with Type 2 diabetes, you are not likely to develop ketosis or ketoacidosis, but your diabetes care professional may recommend a urine ketone test if your blood glucose levels are above normal or when you are sick or under severe stress. The ketone test is available as a tablet or a dip-and-read strip.

Perhaps one of the most important diabetes tests is done in the doctor's office. The test is called a glycosylated hemoglobin (or hemoglobin A1c) assay. It provides a picture of what has been happening over a period of weeks. It tells where your glucose levels have been, on the average, for up to eight to ten weeks before the test.

At-home self blood glucose tests simply show where your glucose levels are at the time of the measurement. The results are vital for any necessary adjustments and for establishing patterns of control, but they are only a snapshot of your blood glucose levels. The results of a hemoglobin A1c test enable the diabetes care professional to chart a long-range management course for you, while you make minor, day-to-day adjustments. The goal for diabetes management is to achieve and maintain a glycosylated hemoglobin level of 7 percent or less.

Currently, this test can be done using tabletop equipment in the doctor's office. Perhaps in the future you will be able to do this test at home with equipment as accurate and reliable as a blood glucose monitor.

Another lab test measures the average blood glucose level for a two-week period. The fructosamine test, marketed under the name RoTag, can by useful when you and your health care provider are making frequent adjustments in your diabetes management plan and want feedback. This test is particularly useful for pregnant women.

Checkup Schedule

Since concerns about health encompass much more than your diabetes, your checkup schedule should consider your entire health. Most of these checks can be done at home. Others are best done by health professionals. Some should be done every day, others less frequently. Here are some suggestions:

Each Day:

- Measure and record your blood glucose levels.
- Make adjustments in your diabetes management plan if the measurements are considerably above, or below, your normal range—or even if they are slightly abnormal at the same time of day for a few days in a row.
- Examine your feet thoroughly. Look for any changes, such as growths, swelling, redness, cuts, or bruises. If you detect a problem, either treat it according to the instructions you've received from your doctor or report it to your doctor.
- Check your sight and the appearance of your eyes. If you notice a change in your vision or an irritation or swelling in the eyes, contact your eye doctor right away.
- Check your skin and treat minor problems such as scratches, cuts, and bruises immediately, based on doctor's instructions.
- Check for chafing and blisters (and start treatment as advised by your doctor). Switch to clothing and socks that won't irritate the affected areas and that will prevent future irritations.
- Eat foods that fit within your diabetes eating plan. Use a diary to record what you eat and when.
- Take the right dosage of medication at the right time. To be sure, use a diary to record when, and how much medication you take.
- If you are scheduled to exercise, follow through on the commitment.

Every Few Days:

- Every seven days, weigh yourself, particularly if you are on a weight-loss or weight-maintenance program. This isn't necessary every day since day-to-day weight fluctuations are normal but can cause anxiety.
- If you have high blood pressure, do a home measurement according to your doctor's recommended schedule.

Every Few Months:
- Check how different foods affect blood glucose levels. Do a blood glucose measurement before you eat a new food and then one hour after. Remember, however, that the results will vary when you combine this food with others that are included in a complete meal.
- Check your exercise equipment to make sure everything is in good working order.
- Check the shoes you wear during exercise to make sure they provide necessary cushioning and support and aren't worn out. Replace or repair anything that is not in top shape.
- Check on your general health and your diabetes health by scheduling a visit with your doctor. Have a hemoglobin A1c test done. If your doctor does not routinely do a hemoglobin A1c test at each visit, request one.

Every Season:
- Adjust activities to the season.
- Protect your skin and eyes from the sun's heat and rays during the summer and the cold and dampness of winter.
- Check your clothes and footwear to be sure they provide proper protection from the weather.
- During winter, look out for excessive skin dryness and cracking. In summer, watch out for rashes that may develop in the moist folds of your skin.
- Use a sunscreen, summer and winter, to protect your skin against burning. A minimum SPF of 15 is recommended.

Once a Year or More:
The following general health checks are recommended for adults, whether or not they have diabetes. The frequency for these examinations depends on your age, sex, and medical/family history.
- Get a comprehensive physical exam, including cardiovascular and comprehensive blood/urine chemistry analysis—including cholesterol and blood lipids.
- Have your blood pressure measured at least once a year; more frequently if high blood pressure is present.

- Have the following examinations at least once a year, or more frequently if you have specific health problems:
  - Colorectal examination (fecal occult blood and/or colonoscopy)
  - Prostate/testicular examination
  - Mammography, Pap smear, and pelvic exams
  - Chest X-ray
  - Dental examination (teeth, gums, oral cavity, with full mouth X-rays)
  - Kidney and liver function tests
  - Eye exams (a must every 12 months for the person with diabetes without eye complications; more frequently when complications are present)
  - Foot examination to check for any nerve damage, changes in the circulation in your feet and legs, or signs of other foot problems, such as corns, calluses, or fungal infections
- Review your prescribed eating plan and evaluate whether any changes are needed. (If necessary, work with a qualified dietitian.)
- Set aside time at least once a year to do a self-examination of your skin—over your entire body. Get completely undressed and stand in front of a full-length mirror in a well-lit area. Look for any changes, such as areas of redness, swelling, or excessively dry patches. Be on the alert for any changes in the size, color, or shape of moles. Use a hand mirror to view more inaccessible areas or get help from someone in your household. If you notice changes, get in touch with your diabetes doctor or dermatologist right away.
- Check the contents of your medicine cabinet. Discard prescription and nonprescription medications that you no longer use or have passed their expiration dates. See that you have adequate and fresh first aid supplies such as adhesive bandages, antibacterial ointment, and alcohol pads. Check to see that your blood glucose monitoring strips are

not beyond their expiration date or have been exposed to excessive moisture or heat. Check to see that your supplies of moisturizing creams, lotions, and sunscreens are adequate. Throw away anything and everything that is old, discolored, out of date, or no longer used.

CHAPTER 10

Sex and Sexuality

ONE OF THE most common concerns of people with diabetes, especially those newly diagnosed, is that it may affect their sex life. Sexuality is an enjoyable part of life, no matter your age. To be fully active sexually depends on many things, including the right attitude and motivation. For people with diabetes, good blood glucose control may also be key, because without good control, all sorts of things can interfere with sexuality.

As with most aspects of sexuality, there are different parameters and potential problems for women and men. But here are some basics that apply to both genders, followed by information specifically for men and for women.

As we said, attitudes have a lot to do with sex and sexuality. What is your attitude toward sexuality? Take inventory. Do you have positive feelings about being a sexy man or woman? Or do you have negative feelings, saying to yourself, "I'm too old for this nonsense?"

Being disturbed by the fact that you have diabetes can interfere with a normal, healthy approach to human sexuality. Perhaps you feel depressed as a result of your diabetes or have begun to experience some diabetes-related complications. If you are depressed, your sex drive and a healthy sexual self-image may suffer—or disappear altogether. Few people get in the mood for enjoyable activities when they are feeling "down."

The passage of time can also influence attitudes toward sexuality. Although birthday celebrations were great fun when we were 21, they seem to lose their thrill with 55 or 60 candles on a cake. And, while many people relish the thought of all that freedom when their last child moves out, they may find it depressing to see an empty bedroom and sit down to a quiet dinner table. As we age, our bodies change, too—usually not for the better, which can also affect attitudes.

Interestingly, attitudes toward sexuality may be influenced by blood glucose levels. Research shows that high blood glucose levels create a sense of hopelessness and helplessness. Such emotions rarely stimulate feelings of positive sexuality.

There is little we can do about aging or the fact that children become adults. But, you are lucky that you can take control of your blood glucose levels and eliminate high blood glucose as a source of trouble. Plus, diabetes management plans feature steps that will improve looks, self image, and sexuality, in addition to diabetes control. Following an eating plan, exercising, keeping blood glucose in good control, and improving your attitude toward life will all contribute to a new positive, sexy self-image.

Of Special Interest to Women
Vaginal Infections

Blood glucose levels that are not in good control place women at increased risk for developing vaginal infections caused by yeast, bacteria, or fungus. If these infections are present, your sex life may become limited because it simply becomes too painful to participate.

Effective and safe medications are available for treating vaginal infections. Some nonprescription medications are even available because this problem is fairly common. Before using an over-the-counter medication, be sure to get your doctor's okay. The newer antifungal drugs may impact the effect of oral hypoglycemic agents. Check with your doctor before you take any medication, prescription or otherwise.

And remember that vaginal infections, like other infections, may not respond to medication if blood glucose levels are above the normal range.

Aging and Menopause

You may find that age and a changing body are affecting your attitude towards sexuality and your physical capabilities. Hormonal changes affecting skin, hair, and nails are common to women during and after perimenopause. The normal aging process is accelerated by cigarette smoking, which also harms blood vessels, nerves, and lungs, and increases the risks for cancer and heart disease. So if you smoke, now's the time to stop.

You can slow some of the effects of aging by keeping in good physical and mental shape, maintaining a positive attitude, and protecting your skin and body from the harmful influences of the sun, excess fat, and inactivity.

Age-related changes occur in all women, but diabetes can speed up the process if blood glucose levels in the normal range are not maintained. Long periods of high glucose levels may interfere with the pituitary gland, the so-called "master" gland that affects most basic body functions. High blood glucose may also interfere with the secretion of the sex hormone estrogen. (In men, high blood glucose levels reduce secretion of the male hormone testosterone.)

Prolonged high blood glucose levels may damage the nerves that stimulate tissues in the vagina, causing a decrease in lubrication and comfort. Nerve damage also can interfere with a woman's ability to experience sexual climax.

Not everything about aging and menopause is negative. One of the good things is that you don't need to worry about birth control anymore. Nor will you be troubled by premenstrual tension or inconvenienced by a monthly period. Still, menopause can create some problems.

At menopause your ovaries stop producing the hormones estrogen and progesterone. When these hormones are not produced, your body's aging process accelerates. Lack of estrogen and progesterone can cause:

• Hair, skin, and nail changes
• Wrinkles
• Hot flashes

- Heart palpitations
- Irritability, anxiety, and sharp swings in mood and emotions
- Bone loss
- Increased risk for heart attacks
- Increased risk for stroke
- Increased levels of blood cholesterol
- Redistribution of body fat stores
- Shrinkage of vaginal tissues
- Loss of vaginal lubrication
- Increase of intercourse-related pain
- Change in response to antidiabetic medication (oral agent or insulin) requiring a change in dosage
- Retention of body fat requiring more effort to lose excess weight

Fortunately, there are effective treatments for perimenopausal problems. Your physician may prescribe one or a combination of two female hormones to replace the loss of naturally produced hormones. If you have a history of breast cancer, endometrial or uterine cancer, or blood clots, you may find that you can't take these hormones without increased risk of side effects. Be sure to discuss this subject in depth with your doctors.

Osteoporosis

Women are at increased risk for osteoporosis once their body stops producing female hormones. Bone density decreases and bones become more brittle and apt to break due to a fall or other accident.

Although some things can be done to strengthen bones when osteoporosis first appears, the best approach to this potentially life-damaging condition is prevention. The idea is to start a preventive program early in a woman's life and continue it as part of a healthy lifestyle.

An osteoporosis prevention program builds on the following list of do's:

I. DO PERFORM WEIGHT-BEARING EXERCISES TO STRENGTHEN YOUR BONES AND MUSCLES. Weight-bear-

A TOUCH OF DIABETES

ing exercises including lifting weights or carrying them as you walk briskly.

2. DO STOP SMOKING. No ifs, ands, or buts.... Just stop!

3. DO STOP OR SIGNIFICANTLY CUT DOWN YOUR IN-TAKE OF CAFFEINE-RICH BEVERAGES. This includes coffee, tea, colas, and even chocolate.

4. DO INCREASE YOUR INTAKE OF CALCIUM by eating or drinking low-fat dairy products. If your eating plan does not permit this, talk to your doctor about taking calcium dietary supplements.

5. DO CONSULT YOUR DOCTOR ABOUT HORMONE RE-PLACEMENT THERAPY when you first notice the signs of menopause. New agents now available come as pills or patches. Dosage can be adjusted to suit your needs and your lifestyle.

(Note that the earlier in life you start this program, the greater the benefits. Still, even if you are past menopause, you can lower some risks by following this program.)

Pregnancy
If you are child-bearing age and want to have a child, the most important thing to do is bring your blood glucose into the normal range and keep it there—both before you try to conceive and throughout your pregnancy and beyond.

There are steps to take while you are working to bring your blood glucose into the normal range. Start a weight-loss diet if necessary and continue (or start) a program of regular exercise. Take medication as needed and monitor your blood glucose frequently. Finally, practice safe and effective birth control methods until your diabetes is in good control and you're ready for a family. The following pages contain information about birth control options and their effects, if any, on diabetes.

Birth Control Options
Hormones

One of the current techniques for birth control uses a combination of female hormones to prevent conception. The most popular form, the oral contraceptive known as "The Pill," is 99 percent effective when used correctly. But while the pill is effective, it does carry the risk of some side effects. These side effects are minimized with the progestin-only oral contraceptive known as the "minipill."

The pill may not be for you if you have a history of heart disease, stroke, high blood pressure, or blood vessel problems such as phlebitis or thrombosis. Health risks increase if you use the pill and smoke. There are many dosage forms and combinations of oral contraceptives available, all by prescription only.

Depo Provera is administered by injection and is active for up to three months. Norplant is a hormone-releasing device that is implanted just beneath the skin of the upper arm. The contraceptive effect of this device is reputed to last up to five years. Even so, Depo Provera and Norplant raise blood glucose and thus are not ideal for women with Type 2 diabetes.

Check with your doctor to find out whether you are a candidate for a hormone-based contraceptive and, if so, which kind is best for you.

The Diaphragm

When fitted properly and used correctly, the diaphragm can be up to 95 percent effective. Its effectiveness increases when used with a spermicidal jelly or foam. Although it has no side effects, the diaphragm requires advance planning for proper insertion before intercourse.

The diaphragm must be fitted by a health care professional who will also teach you how to use it properly.

Condoms

When used properly, condoms may be up to 85 percent effective for birth control. They are more effective when used with a spermicidal jelly or foam. The condom is also an effective barrier to the spread of sexually transmitted diseases. Of course, use of the condom requires the active cooperation of a male partner.

The Sponge
A relatively new birth control device, this sponge-like object contains a spermicidal agent and is placed in the vagina prior to intercourse. The reliability of the sponge has not yet been demonstrated.

The IUD (Intrauterine Device)
Years ago, the IUD was found to be highly effective, but it may carry some health risks, most notably pelvic inflammatory disease (PID). Because the IUD was suspected of causing PID, many manufacturers stopped making this device. However, now two devices appear safe: the copper IUD and the progesterone-treated IUD. Check with your doctor about the availability and suitability of an IUD if you are interested in learning more about it.

Rhythm and Withdrawal
These two methods are the least effective birth-control techniques. The rhythm method means avoiding intercourse around the period of ovulation. The rhythm method is not very reliable, so it is not recommended for women with Type 1 diabetes, who especially need good blood glucose control before becoming pregnant. The withdrawal method also requires precise timing, and is rarely effective.

Permanent Birth Control
If you do not plan to have children, you and your spouse can consider a permanent method of birth control. For men, the surgical technique is called a vasectomy, which works to prevent sperm from being ejaculated. Vasectomies can be performed in a doctor's office under local anesthesia. Vasectomies can be reversed to restore function, but the results are mixed.

For women, the permanent birth control technique is called tubal ligation. The tubes through which the eggs (ova) pass on the way to the uterus are blocked or cut. This procedure is generally done under general anesthesia. You would want, of course, to discuss these options with your physician if you are considering any of these techniques for birth control.

Of Special Interest to Men

Sexuality is a very important part of life for many men. As with women, there are emotional barriers that can hinder sex drive. If you are depressed or angry about having diabetes, your self-image and sexuality will probably suffer.

Your appearance can also affect self-image. So, although you can't stop the passage of time, you can slow down or even reverse some changes to your body.

The first step is learning how to cope with having diabetes and the fact that you need manage it throughout your life. Once you do this, though, you'll gain control and be ready to make changes that will help improve your self-image.

If you're dealing with some extra padding around your waist (larger than love handles) and elsewhere, you can cut down on your calories and increase your physical activity. Reducing calorie intake plus increased physical activity is the best way to lose extra pounds and keep them off for good. You'll look better when you lose extra weight and you'll also feel better about yourself. As an added bonus, losing excess weight is important for getting blood glucose levels into the normal range.

It's vitally important for men with diabetes to get their blood glucose levels within a normal range and keep them there. This kind of blood glucose control should be your immediate goal once you are diagnosed with diabetes. Even if you have had diabetes for a few years and you've not yet reached that goal, now is the time to get started. You lower your risks for major diabetes complications that are exclusive to men when blood glucose is under control. The major complication for men with diabetes is impotence.

Impotence

About 50 percent of men with diabetes between the ages of 30 and 80 become impotent within a decade of being diagnosed with diabetes. That's a frightening statistic. But it is one that may be able to be reduced, since it is based on studies done on men who have had diabetes for more than 10 years.

It has only been within the past decade that the importance of tight blood glucose control was confirmed and the tools to normalize blood glucose have become available.

You can influence the statistical risks for yourself by starting and maintaining a program of tight blood glucose control. That means following your eating plan, losing excess weight if needed, exercising regularly, taking diabetes medication if prescribed, and monitoring blood glucose frequently.

If you are experiencing impotency, meaning you are unable to develop and maintain an erection, you need to determine, with the help of a qualified health professional, whether it is a temporary problem or an ongoing one with emotional or physical causes.

Many men suffer temporary impotency from time to time. Stress, anxiety, a physical illness, and depression are all common causes. An occasional impotency problem is nothing to worry about. However, if the problem occurs regularly, you need to take action.

Don't be ashamed to talk about impotence when you visit your diabetes health care team members. If the problem stems from emotions or attitudes, get psychological counseling and support. Your health care professional can refer you to a therapist. If your problem has a physical basis, which may or may not be related to your diabetes, you may need medical treatment or surgery. You may also need some psychological counseling or support.

If, on the other hand, you experience diabetes-related impotence, the first and most important thing to do is get your blood glucose back into the normal range and keep it there. Prolonged periods of high blood glucose can damage both blood vessels and nerves, and nerve damage is one of the major causes of impotence.

In the male, nerves carry messages from the brain to the penis to tell it the "owner" is aroused. The messages signal the blood vessels, which in turn allow blood to pool in the penis to form the erection. The messages also go to the skin causing an increase in sensitivity and to the muscles to maintain an erection.

These messages travel along nerves to the sexual organs. If these nerves are damaged, the messages can't get through and the penis is unable to react to the arousal stimulus.

When the nerves are not damaged severely, reducing the blood glucose levels can restore normal function. When damage is severe, however, as is the result of prolonged exposure to high blood glucose levels, nerve damage is permanent and irreversible. You will probably be referred to a urologist if this occurs. This specialist can devise a treatment plan that might include using a device or prescription medication. (More information about these treatments follows.)

Doctors take a number of steps to determine the cause(s) of impotence. In all probability, the doctor will check your male hormone levels to determine if they are below normal. If they are, hormone replacement therapy may be prescribed.

Your doctor will also want to know about medications you take in addition to oral hypoglycemic agent or insulin. Some medications, whether prescription or over the counter, can affect your ability to have an erection. If a medication is found to be the culprit, your doctor may be able to change your medication to one with fewer side effects.

You will also be asked about your smoking and drinking habits. Here are some tips:
- If you smoke, stop.
- If you drink more than small amounts of alcoholic beverages, you should cut back.
- Both nicotine and alcohol can affect your ability to have an erection.

MECHANICAL, SURGICAL, AND MEDICAL APPROACHES TO TREATMENT A number of mechanical devices are available that can help you maintain an erection. Some doctors recommend a vacuum erection device, which consists of a plastic cylinder that fits over the penis and a pump that creates a vacuum to help draw blood into the penis. A constricting device is used to keep the blood from flowing out of the penis, also allowing the man to maintain erection.

There are other mechanical devices, but these must be implanted surgically. One device is a penile prosthesis implant that stays rigid; another is an implant that is hooked to a pump.

If the cause of impotence is diagnosed as clogged blood vessels, there is a procedure used to bypass the clogged vessels and increase blood flow to the organ, allowing an erection. Because of the complexity of this procedure, however, it is only used as a last resort.

There are injectable medicines such as yohimbine and the urethral suppository alprostadil (Muse), a prostaglandin derivative that some men find helpful to acquire and maintain an erection. The new oral medication Viagra has proven effective in combating erectile dysfunction. This prescription drug has some side effects, though, and should not be used if you are taking nitroglycerin. And there are a number of other medications in clinical trials that offer promise of help in this medical condition.

If impotence is a problem for you, be sure to discuss it with your doctor. Just remember, getting that blood glucose level under control is the first step toward recovery.

CHAPTER II

Complications

FOR THE PAST DECADE OR SO, doctors and other diabetes health care professionals have been telling patients with diabetes that they may be able to prevent or lessen the severity of diabetes complications if they maintain good blood glucose control. The advice was based on subjective observations of some people who maintained good control and seemed to develop fewer and less severe complications than people who had poor control.

If you heard this 10 years ago, you might not have been impressed. Yes, good control seemed like a good idea, but you wanted facts. Today we have data.

In 1993, the results of the nationwide Diabetes Control and Complications Trial (DCCT) were released. These results showed that tight control can prevent, delay, or reduce the severity of eye, nerve, and kidney complications. The DCCT was begun in the early 1980s to determine whether normalization (or near normalization) of blood glucose levels could help prevent or delay diabetes complications. The trial was also designed to determine whether people with diabetes could achieve and maintain blood glucose levels in the normal to near-normal range.

The study was originally designed to last 10 years, but it ended a year early because the results were so dramatic and positive. Scientists found that people who maintained normal or near-normal blood glucose levels were able to reduce their risks for eye problems by 76 percent, for nerve problems by 60 percent, and for kidney problems by 56 percent, all by having glycosylated hemoglobin levels average less than 7.2 percent.

Information on the reduction of heart disease and stroke were not obtained, but scientists involved in the study said there was "good evidence" that tight control also reduced the risks for these complications.

The DCCT involved people with Type 1 diabetes only. Half these people were placed on what is called an "intensive" therapy program comprised of three or more injections of insulin daily, or use of an insulin infusion pump. The "intensive" therapy was designed to produce normalization of blood glucose levels.

These people adjusted insulin dosage based on four or more blood glucose measurements each day. They also received intensive education on diabetes management (including diet, exercise, and stress management) and maintained close contact (by telephone or in person) with their diabetes health care team. Contact was made at least once each month.

The other half of the study participants remained on a "conventional" management program—one or two insulin injections daily plus some education about diet and nutrition. They monitored their glucose (blood or urine) only once a day and visited their health care team every three months.

The "intensive" therapy team members were the clear winners when it came to preventing or lessening long-term diabetes complications. But what, you must be wondering, does this have to do with you as a person with Type 2 diabetes?

Although you probably will never need to go on "intensive" therapy for Type 2 diabetes, you should maintain good blood glucose control to reduce your risks for diabetes complications. After all, if tight control can do this for people with Type 1 diabetes, it certainly can do this for people with Type 2 diabetes. Here's a step-by-step plan.

Start by tightening up control of your blood glucose levels. If you are monitoring once a day, you may want to take an additional reading during the day. You can stick with your eating plan, maintain your weight-loss and weight-maintenance program, and keep up your physical activity or exercise schedule.

You can also keep in closer touch with your diabetes health care team members, informing them of your progress and any problems, asking questions, and getting new information as it becomes available.

You may also want to change your mind-set about your diabetes and your future. Armed with the facts revealed by the DCCT, you can now trust that your actions to control diabetes will prevent, delay, or reduce the severity of future complications. If you already have some mild complications that haven't yet caused permanent damage, you may be able to use the tight-control program to reverse these effects. In other words, it is never too late to start a program of tight blood glucose control.

You should know that a tight-control program does require an investment of time, effort, and money. It is, however, an investment that pays great dividends if you can avoid hospitalization and expensive medical treatments for a complication, loss of work, pain, inconvenience, loss of vision, impotence, or kidney failure.

At the same time, a tight-control program will put you at risk for some short-term diabetes complications, in particular, low blood glucose. This is because the tighter your control, the greater the risk that your actions will push your blood glucose below your normal range.

On the other hand, if you don't opt for tight control, you are at risk for the short-term complication of hyperglycemia, plus the long-term complications that affect the eyes, nerves, blood vessels, heart, and kidneys.

Short-Term Complications
Low Blood Glucose (also called hypoglycemia or insulin reaction)
Low blood glucose is the most frequent complication experienced by people with diabetes, particularly those who inject insulin, but sometimes it also occurs in those who use an oral hypoglycemic agent. This complication can occur if you skip a meal, exercise too hard or too long, or if you experience severe or prolonged stress.

The risk of having below-normal-range blood glucose levels is reduced for you as a person with Type 2 diabetes instead of Type 1, but it is still present, and you need to know about it and what to do when it occurs.

When blood glucose levels begin to drop below the normal range, you may start to feel uncomfortable, weak, and sweaty. You may also start to act strangely, becoming irritable and irrational. If your blood glucose level continues to fall, you may pass out, go into a coma, and eventually die, unless the low blood glucose is treated properly.

Fortunately, the treatment for low blood glucose is simple: eat or drink a quick-sugar food or beverage, such as a candy, regular soda pop, or glass of orange juice.

When blood glucose drops so low that you pass out, you will need emergency treatment—from a family member or friend first, if possible, then from a medical professional. The emergency medical treatment is usually an injection of the hormone glucagon, which raises blood glucose levels. Many people who have frequent low blood glucose attacks keep a supply of glucagon at home, at the office, or in a small container that they carry with them.

Unfortunately, many people with diabetes do not recognize that their blood glucose levels are becoming low. To overcome this problem, the fastest and most accurate way to determine where your blood levels are is to do a blood glucose measurement whenever you feel "out of sorts." The measurement will take the guesswork out of determining what is causing your symptoms.

Signs and Symptoms of Low Blood Glucose
- Nervous, shaky feeling, and dizziness
- Weakness
- Excessive sweating
- Headache
- Irritability
- Blurred or double vision
- Convulsions
- Loss of consciousness

High Blood Glucose (also called hyperglycemia)

It was undoubtedly hyperglycemia, or high blood glucose, that enabled your doctor to diagnose your diabetes. The diabetes management program that your doctor prescribed for you is most likely designed to reduce above-normal blood glucose levels. If you are successful with your management program, you should be able to significantly reduce the frequency and magnitude of high blood glucose episodes. But you may not be able to eliminate them entirely.

Over long periods, high blood glucose levels are the primary cause of diabetes-related complications discussed throughout these pages. While occasional periods of high blood glucose may make you uncomfortable, they don't pose a serious health threat to those with Type 2 diabetes. This is not the case for people with Type 1 insulin-dependent diabetes because hyperglycemia can lead to a life-threatening condition called ketoacidosis. People with Type 2 diabetes are not prone to this condition, but they may develop its precursor, ketosis.

Ketosis occurs when glucose builds up in the bloodstream but does not reach the cells where it can be used as an energy source. Without glucose, the cells turn to other energy stores, namely fat cells. When cells burn fat as fuel, ketones are formed. These ketones eventually spill out of the body in the urine, where they can be detected with a simple dip-and-read ketone strip. Ketosis can be treated with additional doses of diabetes medication, exercise, treatment of a minor illness, or reduction of stress.

In a roundabout way, the treatment for ketosis points to the possible causes of the high blood glucose levels in the first place. You can send blood glucose levels soaring if you eat too much food, don't exercise enough, have a minor illness, or are under severe stress.

Sometimes, blood glucose levels can jump above normal if you are taking medication for an illness other than diabetes. Sometimes a minor illness alone can elevate blood glucose levels. Sometimes you can prompt hyperglycemia yourself, such as when you start to exercise when your blood glucose levels are already above normal, causing them to soar.

Signs and Symptoms of High Blood Glucose
- Thirst
- Hunger
- Dry mouth
- Frequent urination
- Nausea and vomiting
- Stomach pain
- Deep and rapid breathing
- Unconsciousness (that can lead to coma and death when ketoacidosis goes untreated)

Long-Term Diabetes Complications

Many long-term complications can be prevented, delayed, or minimized in severity when "normal" or near normal blood glucose levels are maintained.

The most frequent long-term complications, their signs and symptoms, and the recommended actions for detecting and treating them are summarized in the following pages.

From Morton's Journal

For most of my life I have been a fatalist. What will be, will be. Diabetes changed all of that.

Once I accepted the fact that I had diabetes, I had to take a close look at my concept of fate, particularly when it comes to viewing what will happen in the future, and specifically when it comes to considering those things over which I have some degree of control.

I know enough about diabetes to know that I can control my future and delay or reduce the severity of complications that result from high blood glucose.

I've read all the studies about the benefits of tight control. I've listened to lectures. I've read (and even written) about how tight control can affect the development of side effects.

I'm not going to gamble on the chance that I am one of those lucky people who never get complications even when they don't bother trying to control blood glucose levels. That's too much of a risk. My brain just won't allow such thoughts to stay in my mind.

I accept the fact that I am not going to be perfect in staying on a diabetes management program. I accept the fact that sometimes my blood glucose levels may be higher than I would like. I don't accept the premise that I am going to automatically develop complications no matter what I do.

Among the good things I do is get regular medical checkups. Right now I am going for a checkup every three months. I feel secure that that sort of monitoring will discover any significant changes or trends, and that I'll be able to take action accordingly.

Actually, if I had to develop a chronic disease, diabetes is certainly tailored for me. I like having the responsibility for following a healthy lifestyle. I like the fact that I am not depending on anyone else to "cure" my disease with a magic pill or shot.

I can take the credit when things go right, and take the blame when they don't.

I like having a good doctor who knows how to diagnose, treat, prescribe, and advise on medical problems. I really like a good diabetes educator who can tell me how to change my lifestyle and who can answer my questions.

Cardiovascular Complications of Type 2 Diabetes

For all of us, greater risks for heart disease, hypertension, strokes, and circulatory problems come as a factor of simple aging. For people with Type 2 diabetes, the risks for these complications are dramatically increased, particularly for someone experiencing weight problems, high blood glucose levels, high blood pressure, and high blood fat levels (cholesterol and triglycerides).

The relationship between cardiovascular disease and diabetes is important:

- People with diabetes have a much higher death rate from cardiovascular disease than people without diabetes. Women without diabetes usually are protected from heart disease until they reach menopause. Women with diabetes seem not to have this protection either before or after menopause.

- People with diabetes have more undiagnosed heart attacks than people without diabetes.
- People with diabetes have an increased risk for heart failure and other cardiac problems than people without diabetes.
- People with diabetes are more apt to develop hypertension than people without diabetes. Untreated hypertension often leads to stroke.
- More people with diabetes suffer from impaired circulation, particularly in the lower legs and feet, than people without diabetes. Impaired circulation can lead to chronic skin ulcers and pain. Untreated, these can develop into gangrene, which is the primary nontrauma-related reason limbs must be amputated.

As with the other long-term complications of diabetes, the most effective approach to dealing with cardiovascular complications is to prevent them. You can do this by following your diabetes eating plan, exercise program, and medication schedule. And, if you are overweight, you need to lose the extra weight and keep it off. Weight loss not only helps control diabetes, it also lowers the risks for future cardiovascular problems.

Not everyone with diabetes confronts the potential complications. Some people are not prone to complications, even if they fail to control their blood glucose levels. On the other hand, some people with diabetes are prone to complications even when they maintain excellent glucose control.

Statistics based on large studies show that 50 percent of men who have had diabetes for 10 years or more are likely to become impotent. This does not mean you will automatically become impotent if you are a male and have had diabetes for 10 years. We know much more about diabetes and how to control it than we used to. If you don't control your blood glucose levels, you may well end up in the half of men who do become impotent.

We now know that if you maintain good control, you can effectively lower the risks of developing any or all of the long-term diabetes complications. Most people don't like to gamble with their health. You are probably no exception. Taking good care of yourself will put you in the good health group statistic.

Frequent Long-Term Diabetes Complications

Background Retinopathy (eyes)
SIGNS AND SYMPTOMS Usually no symptoms are detected

ACTION REQUIRED Have a comprehensive eye exam at least once a year from an eye care professional experienced in diagnosing and treating diabetes-related eye problems.

Proliferative Retinopathy (eyes)
SIGNS AND SYMPTOMS Blurry vision, appearance of floating black spots, appearance of hemorrhages

ACTION REQUIRED Contact eye doctor immediately after experiencing any symptoms. Make adjustments in your diabetes management program to tighten blood glucose control. If needed, have laser treatments to seal leaking blood vessels in the eye.

Nephropathy (kidneys)
SIGNS AND SYMPTOMS Usually no symptoms are detected

ACTION REQUIRED Get a comprehensive medical checkup at least once a year, which includes a urine test for microalbuminuria (an early warning sign of kidney function problems) and a blood pressure measurement. If blood pressure is above normal, follow doctor's recommendation regarding diet, exercise, and use of hypertensive medication. Angiotensin converting enzyme inhibitors (ACE inhibitors) drugs have shown effectiveness in slowing down loss of kidney function. Follow dietary recommendations, which may include salt and protein restrictions. Lose weight if you are carrying excess pounds.

Peripheral Neuropathy (nerves)

SIGNS AND SYMPTOMS Burning, numbness, tingling in feet or hands, hypersensitivity to cold

ACTION REQUIRED Contact doctor immediately when you feel any symptoms. Bring your blood glucose under good control and keep it there. If prescribed, take prescription pain relievers, anti-inflammatory agents, or antidepressants to relieve symptoms. In the future, doctors may prescribe one of the aldose reductase inhibitors currently undergoing clinical evaluation to determine their safety and effectiveness in reversing, preventing, or treating diabetic neuropathy.

Autonomic Neuropathy (nerves)

SIGNS AND SYMPTOMS Impotence, frequent urinary tract infections, inability to fully empty the bladder, bloating, and diarrhea

ACTION REQUIRED Contact your doctor immediately when you become aware of any symptoms. The doctor may prescribe medication to treat urinary infections, combat diarrhea, and aid digestion. Medications and assistive devices are available if impotence is diagnosed as a physical problem. Counseling may be advised if emotional problems are a primary or secondary cause of impotence.

CHAPTER 12

Dear Diary

ONE OF THE BEST TOOLS AVAILABLE to help in diabetes management is a diary. Yes, we are talking about a similar kind of diary people use to record all the significant events of their lives. You may not realize it, but that diary is an excellent companion and friend.

Here are some of the advantages of keeping a diary. It can:

- Enable you to see just how well you are doing to control your blood glucose levels and keep your weight in good control.
- Show patterns in blood glucose control (either above or below normal) that serve as reminders that you should be making adjustments in your management plan.
- Show how your emotions (such as your reaction to stressful events) affect blood glucose levels.
- Show how your body responds to new foods when added to your eating plan.
- Show what weight-loss efforts have done to lower blood glucose levels.
- Show what specific physical activities or exercises do to blood glucose levels.
- Show how a minor illness affects your blood glucose levels.
- Serve as a strong reinforcement for your memory, which begins to function less efficiently as we age.
- Serve as a motivating force to help you stay with the choices you've made for controlling your diabetes.

There are some disadvantages to diary keeping:

- It takes time and effort to record information.
- It may become boring.
- Continuous diary keeping may tempt you to "fudge" your numbers and record activities to make you look good on paper, when in reality, you've been slacking off.
- A diary with inaccurate information can lead diabetes health care providers astray, possibly resulting in missed symptoms leading to future problems.
- A diary may become an unwanted task added to the others required to manage diabetes.
- A diary may be too private to share with your diabetes health care professionals.

Okay, there are the pluses and minuses of diary keeping. If you find the positives outweigh the negatives and think you can benefit from keeping this record, here's a list of basic information you'll want to record, at least as a minimum:

1. The day (one page per day), month, and year.

2. The time(s) and amounts of food you eat (either total calories or exchanges, or breakdown by percentages of fat, protein, and carbohydrates). If you are experimenting with new foods, identify those foods so that you can see what effects they have on your blood glucose levels.

3. Time(s) when you take medications and the type and dosage of the medication.

4. The time(s) and results of self blood glucose measurements. Even if your blood glucose meter has a memory to record the results, it's a good idea to record them in the diary, too.

5. The time(s), duration, and types of physical activity or exercises you do during the day.

6. Any special event in the day, such as illness, vacation, or visits from friends or relatives, especially anything stressful.

7. Your weight as measured at home, particularly if you are on a weight-loss program. Unlike the above information, you should only check your weight once a week, at the same time and under the same approximate conditions (shoes or without, clothed or not). Daily weight checks won't give you accurate information about overall weight loss.

Many people create their own diaries in a notebook and record the above pieces of information. Preprinted diaries are also available, so check your local bookstore or ask your diabetes team or pharmacist for suggestions.

From Morton's Journal

I've opted to do a journal on my computer, rather than use a preprinted diary. Since I'm usually at the keyboard of my computer every day, it's easy for me to open the chapter labeled "Journal" and put my thoughts down on paper (screen/disc).

I also chart my blood glucose readings at the same time I do the journal entry. Even if I don't have anything to write in the journal, the blood glucose measurement, date, and time only take a few seconds of my time. I consider the 30-second reading on the meter I now get a bonus—it gives me an extra 30 seconds to now make an entry in the journal.

I find that writing things down in the journal helps me not only to remember, but it also clarifies my thoughts. It also serves as a Jimminy Cricket conscience—to jog my mind and my body to make some changes when readings are not in the "correct" range, or when journal entries show something significant.

CHAPTER 13

To Learn More About It

ONE OF THE BEST THINGS you can do for yourself is learn all you can about diabetes and diabetes management. Then, keep on learning for the rest of your life!

From Morton's Journal

You can never have too much information. Although my son used to tell me that he couldn't study too long (or too hard) because it may fry his brain, I do think that knowledge is my best weapon against diabetes and, most importantly, against doing things that I know are not good for me. That knowledge may not always stop me from having a martini or a large steak portion, but it will tell me that it's not the end of the world when I do such things—providing I don't make them everyday habits.

I read everything I can get my hands on when it comes to diabetes. I get one journal at home, and avail myself of others during the time I volunteer at the hospital. I read newspapers (two a day) and look for any articles about diabetes. Over the course of the past 30 years, I've had an advantage over most people with diabetes. My work required me to read, to view, to listen, and to discuss diabetes on a full-time basis.

Although I reduced my exposure when I retired, I did not eliminate it. Talking with diabetes educators about new developments has proved to be a valuable asset for me. And attending lectures sponsored by the Diabetes Treatment Center at Sarasota Memorial Hospital helps to refresh my memory as well as to keep me up to date.

Because of my background in the field of diabetes, my doctor is sometimes reluctant to discuss details of the treatment plan. He says, "You know all about these things." Nothing could be further from the truth. I can never know all about diabetes.

The more you know, the better armed you will be to manage not just diabetes, but your entire life. You will make informed choices about your food, your physical activities, and the ways you live your life every day. With up-to-date information, you will minimize guesswork and reduce your chances of mistakes.

You'll also gain independence and freedom by reducing your dependence on family, friends, and health professionals to make your choices. However, this does not mean you'll be working alone to control your diabetes.

You are not alone! You have many resources. You can get information about diabetes from all sorts of resources, including books (you're reading this one, aren't you?), newspapers, magazines, audio and videotapes, and movies. "People" resources might include health professionals—physicians, nurses, dietitians, counselors, and pharmacists.

Your resources can provide information on diabetes in one-to-one counseling sessions or training programs, small or large group seminars, lectures, or training camps. Today you can get interactive information through your computer modem and in the future you may be able to get interactive computer learning programs.

Professional resources are not limited to just individuals trained in diabetes, but include organizations devoted solely to helping people with diabetes. Among these are the American Diabetes Association, Juvenile Diabetes Foundation, and American Association of Diabetes Educators.

Some of the best help may come from people who have diabetes and have learned how to solve certain problems. Many local diabetes organizations, including those based in hospitals, sponsor support groups that meet regularly to discuss diabetes problems and solutions.

Although some resources (the publishers of informational materials, for example) may be headquartered thousands of miles away from your home, you may be able to find other resources in your own town. Even if you live in a rural area, you can establish a communications link with your telephone.

Reading a single book about diabetes and thinking you have completed your diabetes education won't work. Attending a five-session diabetes education program at your hospital does not do the whole job, either. You will want to get information from many sources and keep updated on emerging information.

Science is progressing so rapidly in its quest to gain knowledge that what was considered current in this year will become obsolete or perhaps incorrect two years from now. You need to stay abreast of scientific progress to keep your own diabetes management program current.

The bottom line is that your personal diabetes education program needs to be lifelong. Just read the following developments we've seen in diabetes in the last two to three years.

Tight control of blood glucose can prevent, delay, or minimize many of the key complications of diabetes.

Tight control requires strict adherence to a recommended management program that may include multiple insulin injections and certainly requires frequent blood glucose measuring. Adjustments to individual management programs are made daily based on test results. The program also requires close and frequent communication between the person with diabetes and members of his or her health care team.

It is okay for a person whose diabetes is in good control to eat a little bit of sugar as part of a well balanced meal.

Many with diabetes have been told for years that any sugar at all was forbidden. Recently, though, nutritional research has revealed that a person with diabetes can consume some treats containing sugar. There are some provisions: blood glucose must be in good control and the sweet treat must be part of a well balanced meal (not eaten alone as a snack, which can cause harmful blood glucose spiking).

Mild to moderate physical activities for only 10 minutes, three to four times a day provide the same benefits as working out at some organized exercise for 30 minutes, three to four times a week.

Your choices are greatly expanded by this relatively new scientific finding. You can take a 10-minute walk after each meal to fulfill your exercise requirement, mow the lawn, do housework, clean the garage, or walk up and down the aisles of the local market. You don't have to join a health club or buy special exercise clothing or equipment.

Some of those things we can take for granted today were considered forbidden in diabetes management just a few years ago or not even considered. Self blood glucose monitoring was not available in 1980. From 1945 to 1980, the only kind of self-test was urine sugar testing.

In the decade before the first urine sugar test was developed, a person with diabetes had to use a Bunsen burner, teaspoon, and a reagent powder to test urine to see if sugar was present. Needless to say, this was less than accurate.

The development of the blood glucose reagent strip and the portable blood glucose meter radically changed the approach to self management for people with diabetes.

For those who need insulin, scientists have in the last 15 years developed techniques allowing manufacturers to produce "human" insulin. Human insulin became the medication of choice for people who require insulin injections because it lowered the risk of allergic response and resistance to animal source insulin. In addition, there are now insulin analogs, so-called designer insulins, to give the person with diabetes even more options.

For people with Type 2 diabetes, the introduction of second generation hypoglycemic agents has been good news. These carry a lower risk of side effects than the original version and may even be more effective. Subsequent generations are likely to prove even better, so stay tuned.

In the field of nutrition, there have been many changes in the last few years. Not long ago, people with diabetes were advised to fast to control their diabetes. Later, the diabetes eating plan was based on a high-fat, low-carbohydrate formula. Within the past 15 years, the high-carbohydrate, high-fiber diet was deemed best for people with Type 2 diabetes.

Today, some scientists are questioning the benefits of a high-carbohydrate diet and recommend instead a well balanced diet for everyone, not just for people with diabetes. Some extol the virtues of monounsaturated fat, such as from olive oil, and warn against polyunsaturated fats. All seem to agree, however, that saturated fat can be harmful.

A short time ago, nutritionists touted the benefits of fish oil in the diet. But recent studies have shown that fish oil in the quantities obtained when fish is eaten five to six times per week as part of a regular eating plan shows no effect over a non-fish eating plan.

If your diabetes education took place a decade or so ago, we hope you have kept abreast of the scientific and medical developments that have occurred. Medical and scientific research is moving forward at an ever-increasing speed. In the future, the information superhighway will serve to speed the dissemination of vital data. Indeed, there are many Internet locations already available for computer users with diabetes.

Where to Go

After you choose to learn all you can about diabetes, your first step may be to ask your doctor or the office nurse about resources available to you in your community. There may be a local chapter of the American Diabetes Association (ADA). The ADA maintains a library of educational materials and sponsors educational courses, monthly meetings and activities such as lectures, and support groups.

There may also be a diabetes center at the local hospital or community center where educational courses on various diabetes subjects are available. Perhaps one-to-one sessions on diabetes and nutrition, and training programs on the latest in self blood glucose monitoring are offered.

Both the community center and the hospital's diabetes center may sponsor support groups for people with Type 2 diabetes who have interests and challenges similar to yours. Use the local telephone directory to find out how to contact them.

The phone book is a good source in itself for finding resources. The white pages lists names, addresses, and phone numbers of private organizations such as the ADA. The blue pages lists information on governmental organizations like the Council on Aging, Medicare, and Medicaid.

Other places to get information include libraries and bookstores. You'll find a variety of books on diabetes—some written by experts, others by people who have faced the same management challenges you face and have learned various approaches to diabetes.

Many books provide basic, helpful information. There are books on exercise and how to cope and live with diabetes. There are also cookbooks with recipes tailored to diabetes eating plans.

Be sure to check the dates of publication. With the body of knowledge about diabetes changing so rapidly, there's bound to be out-of-date information out there. Be sure your resources are as current as possible. A few basic books, including the ADA exchange lists and some cookbooks, may be all you really need to own.

Your local ADA office can provide a listing of books, booklets, films, and videos that can be ordered from ADA headquarters. Other resources for printed material include your doctor's office and the hospital where pamphlets are generally available at no cost.

Some booklets give an overview of diabetes in fairly simple language; others concentrate on a single subject, such as self blood glucose monitoring. Many of these free pamphlets are published by the manufacturers of diabetes products and supplies.

If you don't find what you need locally, here's a list of national organizations, including Internet E-mail addresses, and support lines that may help you to learn more about your disease.

American Diabetes Association (ADA)
National Service Center
1660 Duke Street
Alexandria, VA 22314

1-800-ADA-DISC

Juvenile Diabetes Foundation (JDF)
120 Wall Street, 19th Floor
New York, NY 10005

1-800-223-1138

American Association of Diabetes Educators (AADE)
444 N. Michigan Ave., Suite 1240
Chicago, IL 60611

1-800-338-3633
1-800-TEAM-UP-4 (for a referral to a local diabetes educator)

National Diabetes Information Clearinghouse
Box NDIC
Bethesda, MD 20892

1-301-468-2162

International Diabetes Center (IDC)
3800 Park Nicollet Blvd.
St. Louis Park, MN 55416

1-612-993-3393

Joslin Diabetes Center
1 Joslin Place
Boston, MA 02215

1-617-732-2415

Diabetes Information on the Internet

At the time of this writing, there were more than 3.75 million pages on the Internet that mentioned the term *diabetes*. There are home pages that present up-to-date medical information. There are pages that deal with diabetes management. There are sites where you can exchange information with other people who have diabetes. There are support groups, chat groups, bulletin boards, and on-line education sessions. If you have a computer, you can access these diabetes-related pages at home. If you don't have a computer, your local library probably has a computer through which you can access the Internet.

Once you get on the Internet, you can let your fingers do the walking by using one of the search engines (Excite, Yahoo, Infoseek, etc.) to find pages that mention diabetes, diabetes management, or any specific subject you are interested in (such as hyperglycemia or neuropathy). Or you can take the easy way out and go to one or more of the major Internet resources.

One of the best is <diabetes.com>, a comprehensive diabetes website that contains excellent diabetes news and information. <Diabetes.com> also provides you with contact with other people with diabetes to discuss your problems, solutions, questions, and answers.

An excellent source for finding diabetes websites, mailing lists, and support groups is <mendosa@mendosa.com>.

<DiabetesMonitor.com> also provides a comprehensive diabetes registry of diabetes websites.

For more scientific information, you can go to <Mediconsult.com>.

A few years ago, the available listings for diabetes totalled 100 or so. Today they are nearing 4 million. By the time you read this book, there will be many, many more. That's why it's a good idea to first go to the sites that list resources (and are most recently updated) or use one of the search engines to find the most current listings.

Magazines and Newsletters

Although magazines and newsletters don't always give in-depth information, you'll want the news they transmit in research and management to stimulate your interest and keep you current. There are many newsletters to choose from. One source might be your local diabetes organization or the ADA state affiliate, which usually provides a periodical when you join.

When you join the ADA, you will get a subscription to a monthly magazine called *Forecast*. This informative publication includes answers to questions, updates on medical advances, and feature stories about people with diabetes.

Another nationally distributed magazine is called *Diabetes Self-Management*. While it is not affiliated with any specific diabetes organization, it publishes a wide variety of articles on diabetes management. It is published every other month by R. A. Rapaport Publishing, Inc. 150 W. 22nd Street, New York, NY 10011. Contact the publisher for subscription rates.

The JDF and the National Diabetes Information Clearinghouse publish either magazines or newsletters. Contact them for specifics.

Recommended Books for your Home Library

Here's a brief list of books that you may want to consider for your personal bookshelf.

Diabetes 101: A Pure and Simple Guide for People Who Use Insulin by Betty Page Brackenridge, M.S., R.D., C.D.E, and Richard O. Dolinar, M.D. A practical and understandable guide if you want to learn more about insulin-dependent diabetes.

Carbohydrate Counting Cookbook by Tami Ross, R.D., C.D.E., and Patti Geil, R.D., C.D.E. A step-by-step introduction to carbohydrate counting, plus 125 recipes based on the meal-planning system.

60 Days of Low-Fat, Low-Cost Meals in Minutes by M.J. Smith, R.D. Over 150 recipes and complete menus for days and more for breakfasts, lunches, dinners, and snacks. Each recipe features complete nutrition analysis, including exchanges.

366 Low-Fat Brand-Name Recipes in Minutes by M.J. Smith, R.D. A year's worth of healthy and fast family favorites using the country's most popular brand-name foods. Each recipe features complete nutrition analysis, including exchanges.

Skim the Fat by the American Dietetic Association. A definitive guide to reducing fat in everything you eat—without sacrificing taste—and maintaining a healthy lifestyle. It includes simple and innovative low-fat cooking techniques and tips for recipe makeovers.

The Diabetes Self-Care Method by Charles M. Peterson, M.D., and Lois Jovanovic-Peterson, M.D. A comprehensive guide to managing your diabetes.

The Diabetic Woman by Lois Jovanovic-Peterson, M.D., June Biermann, and Barbara Toohey. Address the unique problems diabetes creates for women regarding puberty, menstruation, pregnancy, and marriage.

Hormones: The Woman's Answerbook by Lois Jovanovic-Peterson, M.D., and Genell Subak-Sharpe. A guide to understanding women's hormones, including findings on menopause, PMS, and more.

Glossary of Diabetes Terms

GLUCAGON A hormone produced by the pancreas that helps sugar (glucose) stored in the liver to move into the bloodstream. This transfer of glucose into the bloodstream raises blood glucose levels. Injections of commercially manufactured glucagon can help counteract a severe low blood glucose attack, otherwise known as hypoglycemia or insulin reaction.

GLUCOSE The basic form of sugar, glucose provides the fuel necessary for body tissues and organs to function properly. It is the main source of energy to maintain bodily functions. Glucose is the end product of the digestion of foods—proteins, fats, and carbohydrates (including other, more complex sugars such as fructose and sucrose). This glucose circulates in the bloodstream and then enters the body's cells where it is burned as fuel. In order to enter these cells, glucose requires the help of insulin. When there is not enough insulin present, glucose stays in the bloodstream, building up in quantity, and then spilling out through the kidneys into the urine.

GLYCOSYLATED HEMOGLOBIN This type of hemoglobin is also called hemoglobin A1c. Hemoglobin is one of the components of the red blood cells in your bloodstream. Glycosylated hemoglobin is a special molecule that has glucose attached to it.

The number of glycosylated hemoglobin molecules in a specific amount of blood provides information about the average blood glucose levels that have occurred in the person's body during the past six to eight weeks. This average can be determined because individual red blood cells have a short life span of 120 days and the cells that contain glycosylated hemoglobin exist only for this period.

The target level for glycosylated hemoglobin is expressed as 7 percent or less. Any reading above that indicates that the average blood glucose levels during the previous six to eight weeks were above normal.

At the present time, this test can only be done in the doctor's office or in a laboratory. It is hoped that an accurate and easy to use home test may become available in the future.

The glycosylated hemoglobin test is intended to supplement, not replace, the daily self blood glucose measurements. Your measurements tell what your blood glucose levels are at the time of the test. You can then take immediate action by adjusting parts of your diabetes management plan to counteract a too-high or too-low blood glucose level. The glycosylated hemoglobin test cannot do this.

HYPERGLYCEMIA This is the technical term for high blood glucose levels—above 126 mg/dL (fasting) or above 150 to 180 mg/dL (random). Or, above 7 mmol/L (fasting) or above 8.3 to 10 mmol/L (random).

These are arbitrary numbers that apply to the population of people with diabetes as a whole. You and your doctor may consider that a random measurement of 150 mg/dL (8.3 mmol/L) is normal for you, not high. It's best that you establish a normal range with your doctor and consider any readings above or below your normal range to signal a need for action.

This action, in the form of adjustments in your diabetes management plan, should be initiated if you feel symptoms of high blood glucose and confirm these symptoms with a blood glucose measurement.

Generally, the symptoms of hyperglycemia include fatigue, frequent urination, and excessive thirst. But these symptoms can also be present because you have not had enough sleep, if you have consumed too much liquid refreshment, or if you have eaten very salty foods. That's why it's best to do a blood glucose measurement when you suspect something might not be quite right in your body.

If you allow your blood glucose levels to stay moderately high over a period of years, you will increase your risks, significantly, for the development of major complications including retinopathy, neuropathy, and nephropathy.

If you allow your blood glucose levels to go very high, even for a short period, you may develop a condition called ketosis (see page 149).

Although people with Type 2 diabetes are not prone to developing ketoacidosis, the next stage, you may still be at risk. Untreated ketosis can develop into ketoacidosis, which can then cause you to fall into a coma. If this coma and the underlying high blood glucose problem is not treated promptly and properly, death may occur. Emergency hospitalization is usually required.

HYPERTROPHY This is a condition that may develop in persons who inject insulin, but who do not rotate injection sites regularly. The skin around the overused injection site becomes thickened and puffy. Because of this damage to the tissue, the absorption rate of insulin injected into this site may be slowed down.

HYPOGLYCEMIA Low blood glucose, or hypoglycemia (also known as insulin reaction), is at the other end of the spectrum of blood glucose levels from hyperglycemia. Low blood glucose is considered to be any level below 60 to 80 mg/dL (3.3 to 4.4 mmol/L). You may develop low blood glucose if you skip a meal, if you exercise too much, or if you take an improper amount of your diabetes medication.

You may or may not be able to detect the symptoms of low blood glucose. These symptoms may be strong or they may be weak. They may even be nonexistent. But if you feel dizzy or suddenly irritable, if you develop a headache, or if you start to act "funny" according to those around you, you may need to check your blood glucose.

If the measurement confirms that your blood glucose levels have dropped below your normal range, then you need to take action. Action includes eating a snack, drinking a soft drink, eating candy, or taking a glucose tablet or gel to bring glucose levels back up.

Blood glucose levels can drop below normal slowly or very rapidly. There's really no accurate way to predict how your body will handle a low blood glucose reaction. When blood glucose levels drop very low, you are liable to lose consciousness. At that time, you'll need a friend or family member to administer a quick-sugar source to you.

INSULIN Insulin is a hormone secreted by the beta cells in your pancreas gland. This hormone helps the glucose from your bloodstream to enter your body's cells, where the glucose is "burned" as fuel.

In Type 1 diabetes, the beta cells do not produce any insulin. In Type 2 diabetes, the beta cells do produce insulin, but either your body has a resistance to the hormone, which does not allow it to function properly, or the beta cells are producing too little insulin to handle proper amounts of glucose.

Today, the insulin produced commercially in North America is "human" insulin, either manufactured through genetic engineering or partially synthesized. Prior to the development of human insulin, the pancreas glands of pigs and beef cattle were used as sources for this hormone.

Currently, insulin must be injected into the body, either by needle and syringe, by spray injector, or by an insulin infusion pump. Scientists are working on methods to encapsulate insulin so that it may be taken orally and not be destroyed by digestive juices. Science is also working to perfect a form of insulin that may be sprayed into the nostrils or through the mouth and on an insulin pump that can be surgically implanted under the skin.

INSULIN-DEPENDENT DIABETES MELLITUS (IDDM or Type 1 Diabetes) Years ago the terms "Youth-Onset" or "Juvenile Diabetes" were also used to describe this kind of diabetes.

Type 1 diabetes is believed to be an autoimmune disease and, in many people, is an inherited condition. In this form of the disease, the beta cells within the pancreas gland no longer produce any insulin. Because of this, the person with Type 1 diabetes requires injections of insulin in order to stay alive.

The destruction of beta cells may be triggered by a common virus, such as the one that causes mumps. This virus stimulates the body's immune system to release antibodies to destroy the virus. But, because of a genetic defect, the immune reaction process fails to shut down when all of the virus is destroyed. Instead, the body's antibodies target the insulin-producing beta cells in the pancreas and, over a period of years, gradually destroy all of them.

Type 1 diabetes usually, but not always, strikes youngsters from ages 1 through 20 years old.

KETOSIS/KETOACIDOSIS Ketosis is a complication of diabetes that occurs when the body is not able to use (burn) glucose for energy and must use stored fat for fuel instead. In the process of burning fat, ketones are released and then excreted through the body into the urine. A simple urine tablet or strip test can detect the presence of ketones.

Ketones can be detected when blood glucose levels are very high. They can also be present if the person is on a very low-calorie weight-loss diet where the objective may be to burn up excess fat. In people with Type 1 diabetes, however, untreated ketosis may develop into ketoacidosis, a serious condition that can lead to coma and death.

LIPOATROPHY Lipoatrophy is a condition that occurs in a person who injects insulin but does not rotate injection sites. The overused injection site becomes indented and looks like a hollow spot on the skin.

NEPHROPATHY This is a major complication of diabetes that can result from prolonged high levels of blood glucose. In nephropathy, the kidneys cannot filter harmful wastes out of the bloodstream into the urine. This kidney failure is gradual and eventually develops into end-stage kidney failure, which requires dialysis or a kidney transplant to sustain life.

The early stages of nephropathy may be detected by a urine strip test for microalbuminaria. Treatment at this time consists of tight blood glucose control plus a diet restricting intake of proteins.

NEUROPATHY This is one of the most common complications of diabetes. Prolonged periods of high blood glucose levels eventually damage the nerves in various parts of the body. Tight blood glucose control can prevent this complication from occurring, or it can delay and lessen the severity of it. Even when symptoms appear, tight blood glucose control may alleviate symptoms and reverse some of the damage.

There are two forms of neuropathy:

Peripheral neuropathy affects the motor/sensory nerves. These are the nerves that control the muscles in your body. This type of neuropathy causes pain, tingling in the feet, legs or hands, and loss of the ability to sense damage, such as a nail puncture in the sole of the foot or a burn on the skin of an affected hand. In addition to tight blood glucose control, the treatments for peripheral neuropathy may be the use of pain-killing medications and prescription antidepressant drugs. Scientists are working on a class of drugs called aldose reductase inhibitors, which may prove of benefit in the treatment of neuropathy.

Autonomic neuropathy affects the involuntary nerves. These nerves regulate body functions such as digestion or breathing. It may also affect the normal functions of the stomach, the bladder, the genitals, or the heart.

NONINSULIN-DEPENDENT DIABETES (NIDDM or Type 2 Diabetes) This type of diabetes was previously known as "Adult Onset" or "Maturity Onset Diabetes." It is the most common form of diabetes and affects 85 percent of all the people with diabetes. It usually, but not always, develops in people who are over the age of 40. It is being increasingly recognized in younger persons and even children.

Many of the adults who get Type 2 diabetes are overweight or obese. Many of these adults also have blood relatives who also have or had Type 2 diabetes. Women who have Type 2 diabetes may have had children who weighed more than 9 pounds at birth.

Women who have Type 2 diabetes may also have had a type of diabetes called gestational diabetes when they were pregnant. After giving birth, these women saw the gestational diabetes disappear, but years later Type 2 diabetes developed.

Some of the people with Type 2 diabetes were diagnosed as having "Impaired Glucose Tolerance" years before Type 2 diabetes developed. This condition formerly was called borderline diabetes.

In a person with Type 2 diabetes, the beta cells in the pancreas still produce insulin. Sometimes the cells just don't produce enough insulin to handle the glucose in the bloodstream. Sometimes the beta cells produce insulin in sufficient quantities, but the body develops a resistance to this insulin and interferes with insulin's ability to get glucose from the bloodstream into the cells. In either case, the end result is excess glucose in the bloodstream that can't be used as fuel by the body's cells.

Type 2 diabetes can be immediately treated by adopting a lifelong management plan including following a healthful eating plan and building physical activity or exercise into a regular lifestyle. If the person is overweight, then an eating plan will be designed to restrict calorie intake at the same time as it balances nutrients. This balance is usually comprised of large amounts of carbohydrates, medium amounts of protein, and small amounts of fat, plus fiber, vitamins, and minerals.

This approach to treatment can produce almost a total relief from diabetes symptoms if the person sticks to the eating plan and keeps up with the exercise program, and if the overweight person loses excess weight and keeps it off. This requires self-motivation and discipline on the part of the person with Type 2 diabetes.

If the diet and exercise approach does not work, and if blood glucose levels remain above normal, then a diabetes medication may be added to the plan. For many people, this medication will be one of the oral hypoglycemic agents. For some, this medication will be injected insulin, however, and for others there may be a combination of oral agent and injected insulin.

No matter what method of treatment is used to control Type

2 diabetes, the person with this disease needs to monitor blood glucose levels to determine whether or not the plan is working and if adjustments need to be made. Usually, the members of the diabetes health care team and the person with Type 2 diabetes will jointly determine the schedule and frequency of blood glucose measurements.

ORAL HYPOGLYCEMIC AGENTS The oral agent family of medications now consists of a number of medications with different characteristics. They vary in terms of how quickly they act, how long they act, and how often during the day the person must take them.

Oral agents are not insulin. They are medications that help the body to better utilize the insulin it produces and thus help to lower blood glucose levels. Over a period of years, the effectiveness of one oral agent may wear off and the person taking that agent may have to increase dosage or switch to another medication as directed by the physician. For some who experience a "failure" or intolerance with oral agents, injected insulin may be required to maintain control of blood glucose.

RENAL THRESHOLD This is the "spill point," the level at which excess glucose in the blood starts to spill from the kidneys into the urine. The average renal threshold is a glucose level between 160 and 180 mg/dL (8.9 and 10 mmol/L). This spill point can vary with the individual and is usually affected by the age of the person.

Because the exact renal threshold for each individual is unknown, the old-fashioned urine sugar test often produced inaccurate estimates of the actual blood glucose levels at the time of the measurement. That's why the urine sugar test has been replaced by the blood glucose measurement.

RETINOPATHY This is another of the major complications of diabetes and the result of prolonged levels of above-normal blood glucose. Tight blood glucose control can prevent, delay, lessen the severity of, and even reverse the damage caused by diabetic retinopathy, if permanent damage has not yet occurred.

Retinopathy occurs when the small blood vessels in the back of the eye (the retina) are damaged by exposure to high levels of glucose. This damage can result in blurry or impaired vision and blindness.

There are two types of retinopathy:

Background retinopathy involves leakage of fluid from the small blood vessels in the retina. Vision becomes blurred when this occurs. The leaks in the blood vessels can be sealed by laser beam therapy.

Regular eye examinations by an ophthalmologist experienced in the diagnosis and treatment of diabetic eye disease is recommended since early detection can prevent background retinopathy from progressing to the next, more serious stage.

Proliferative retinopathy occurs when background retinopathy goes undiagnosed and untreated, and when blood glucose control continues to be poor.

In this condition, there is growth of fragile, abnormal blood vessels in the retina. These abnormal blood vessels may leak fluid and blood into the eye and interfere with vision. Scarring on the surface of the retina may result, further damaging vision and eventually causing total loss of vision in the affected eye.

While laser beam treatment may be able to seal leaks, once scarring occurs the damage is permanent. As with the early stages of retinopathy, however, tight blood glucose control can slow down progression of this diabetes complication.

Bibliography

Monographs and Books

1. Jovanovic L: *Your guide to a healthy, happy pregnancy.* Biodynamics, Indianapolis, 1981, revision, 1985.

2. Jovanovic L, Braun C, Druzin M, Peterson CM: *The physicians manual: Management of the pregnant diabetic woman.* Biodynamics, Indianapolis, 1981, revision, 1985.

3. Jovanovic L: Practical guide to the management of gestational diabetes, Biodynamics, 1985.

4. Peterson CM, Jovanovic L (eds): *The Diabetes Self Care Method.* Simon and Schuster, New York, 1984. Revised in 1990 and now published by Lowell House, Los Angeles. (Translated into Italian by Geo Publishers, 1992)

5. Peterson CM, Jovanovic L: *A Primer for Glycosylated Hemoglobins.* Helena Laboratories, Beaumont, Texas, 1984.

6. Jovanovic L, Peterson CM (eds): *Contemporary Issues in Nutrition: Diabetes Mellitus,* Alan Liss, New York, 1985.

7. Jovanovic L, Peterson CM (eds): *Diabetes in Pregnancy: Teratology, Toxicology, and Treatment.* Praeger, Philadelphia, 1986.

8. Subak-Sharpe GJ, Jovanovic L, Peterson CM: *Living with Diabetes.* Doubleday and Company, Garden City, New York, 1985.

9. Jovanovic L: *Primary Therapy with Glipizide: A Clinical Report.* Pfizer, Inc., 1985.

10. Jovanovic L and Subak-Sharpe GJ: *Hormones: The Woman's Answer Book,* Atheneum Publishers, NY, 1987. (Translated into French, German, and Canadian English and British English).

11. Jovanovic L, Toohey B, Bieman J: *The Diabetic Woman.* Jeremy Tarcher Publishers, Los Angeles, 1987.

12. Jovanovic L (ed): *Controversies in the Field of Pregnancy and Diabetes.* Springer-Verlag. New York, 1988.

13. Peterson CM, Jovanovic L, Formby B (eds): *Fetal Islet Transplantation as a Treatment of Type I Diabetes Mellitus.* Springer-Verlag, 1988.

14. Jovanovic L, Stone ML, Gabbe SG: *Pregnancy and Diabetes,* Diabetes Treatment Centers of America, March, 1988.

15. Dranov P: *Diabetes: A Random House Personal Medical Handbook.* With a foreword by Lois Jovanovic-Peterson, MD. Random House, New York, 1990.

16. Lodewick P, Bierman J, Toohey B. *The Diabetic Man.* With a foreword by Lois Jovanovic-Peterson, MD. Lowell House, Los Angeles, 1991.

17. Jovanovic-Peterson L, Peterson CM, Stone MB. *A Touch of Diabetes,* Chronimed Publishing, 1991. Second Edition, 1996.

18. Jovanovic-Peterson L, Abrams R, and Coustan DR, Guest Editors. "Gestational Diabetes: Strategies for Management." *Diabetes Spectrum* 5:18–53,1992.

19. Jovanovic-Peterson L, Levert S. *A Woman Doctor's Guide to Menopause.* Hyperion New York, 1993, revised 1996.

20. Jovanovic-Peterson L, Editor-in-Chief. *Medical Management of Pregnancy Complicated by Diabetes.* American Diabetes Association, Inc., Alexandria, VA, 1993, revised 1995.

21. Jovanovic-Peterson L, Williams B, Bevier W, Ahmadizadeh I. *Detecting Diabetic Retinopathy: A Training Guide for Primary Care Providers Developed by The Santa Barbara Diabetes Project.* Canon, Inc., 1993.

22. Bierman J, Toohey B. *The Diabetic Book: All Your Questions Answered,* Third Edition. With a foreword by Lois Jovanovic-Peterson, MD. Jeremy Tarcher Publishers, Los Angeles, 1994.

23. Jovanovic-Peterson L, Stone MB. *Gestational Diabetes.* Chronimed Publishing, 1994.

24. Jovanovic-Peterson L, Peterson CM (eds). *Endocrine Disorders of Pregnancy, Endocrine Clinics of North America.* WB Saunders, Philadelphia, 1995.

25. Peterson CM, Jovanovic-Peterson L, Formby B (eds). *Fetal Islet Transplantation,* Plenum, New York, 1995.

26. Jovanovic-Peterson L (Editor-in-Chief). *Diabetes & Pregnancy: What to expect.* First edition, 1987, second edition, 1990, third edition, 1995. American Diabetes Association, Alexandria, Virginia, 1995, and *Gestational Diabetes: What to expect,* revised 1997.

27. Jovanovic-Peterson L, Biermann J, Toohey B. *The Diabetic Woman,* Revised and Expanded. GP Putman's Sons, New York, 1996.

28. Jovanovic L and Arsham G. *Diabetes Spectrum: From Research to Practice: Diabetes in Women and Men.* American Diabetes Association, Alexandria, VA, 1998.

Index

A

acarbose, 78, 81
ACE inhibitors, 89
Acetohexamide, 76, 80
acupuncture, 39
aerobic exercise, 70
alcohol
   food choices and, 48–49
alpha blockers, 89–90
alpha-glucosidase inhibitors, 78
alprostadil, 119
Amaryl, 76, 80
American Association of Diabetes Educators
   addresses and phone numbers for, 141
American Diabetes Association, 139
   addresses and phone numbers for, 141
   nutrition guidelines for diabetes, 45–49
anaerobic exercise, 70
arthritis medication, 91–92
attitude adjustment, 39–41
autonomic neuropathy, 150
Avandia, 79

B

background retinopathy, 129, 153

beta blockers, 90

biguanides, 77

biofeedback, 38

birth control options, 114–116

    condoms, 114–115

    diaphragm, 114

    hormones, 114

    IUD, 115

    permanent, 115–116

    The Pill, 114

    rhythm, 115

    sponge, 115

    withdrawal, 115

blood glucose levels, 31. *See also* glucose

    colds/illness and, 31

    eating food and, 30

    emotions and, 36

    exercise and, 30–31

    fasting plasma level for diagnosis, 12

    food choices and speed to convert to, 43

    high levels, 32–33

    impotency and, 117–118

    insulin injections and, 31

    low levels, 31–32

    normal range for, 96

    oral hypoglycemic agent, 31

    pre-meal level and insulin injections, 86

    sexuality and, 110

    stress and, 31, 36

    tight control of, and complications, 97–98

blood glucose monitoring

    advances in equipment for, 94, 97

    converting results from mg/dL to mmol/L, 95

    exercise and, 67, 101

    historical background of, 138

    how to, 99

importance of, 94

limitations of, 102

normal range for, 96

pattern of above/below normal measurements, 95

reasons for, 94–95

schedule for, 100

stress and, 101

tight control of blood glucose levels and complications,
  97–98

weight loss and, 101–102

borderline diabetes, 23, 151

C

calorie/fat counting system
  advantages of, 54

calories
  burned by physical activities, 73

  figuring percentage of calories from fat, 57

carbohydrate counting, 52–53
  advantages of, 52–53

  soluble fiber, 53

carbohydrates
  food choices and, 47–48

  in kickoff eating plan, 50

cardiovascular complications, 127–129

cataracts, 33

checkup schedule, 103–107
  each day, 104

  every few days, 104

  every few months, 105

  every season, 105

  once a year or more, 105–107

Chlorpropamide, 76, 80

cholesterol, 47, 90

cholesterol medication, 90–91

circulatory problems
    as complication of diabetes, 127–129
cold medication, 92
colds
    blood glucose levels and, 31
complications
    cardiovascular, 127–129
    high blood glucose, 125–126
    long-term, 126–130
    low blood glucose, 123–125
    nephropathy, 129–130
    retinopathy, 129
    short-term, 123–126
    tight control of blood glucose levels and, 97–98
    Type 1 diabetes, 24
    Type 2 diabetes, 26
condoms, 114–115
cookbooks, 61, 143–144
cough medication, 92

D

Depo Provera, 114
Diabeta, 76, 81
diabetes
    gestational, 23, 26, 151
    heredity and, 44
    historical perspective on, 19–21
    myths about, 12, 26–27
    noninsulin-dependent, 150–152
    risk factors for, 44
    terms for, 23
    Type 1, 23–24, 148–149
    Type 2, 24–26, 150–152
Diabetes Control and Complications Trial, 20, 121–122
    results of, 98
    study groups for, 122

diabetes management program
  benefits of, 13
  historical perspective on, 19–21
  owning responsibility for, 12–13
  for Type 1 diabetes, 24
  for Type 2 diabetes, 25–26
diabetes mellitus, 19
Diabetes Self-Management, 143
diabetic neuropathy, 32
Diabinese, 76, 80
diagnosis
  new criterion for, 12
  reaction to, 11, 35
diaphragm, 114
diary
  advantages of, 131
  disadvantages of, 132
  for exercise, 67
  list of basic information to record in, 132–133
Dymelor, 76, 80

E

eating plan
  best for diabetes, 139
  calorie/fat counting system, 53–54
  carbohydrate counting, 52–53
  cookbooks for, 61
  eating out, 60
  exchange system, 52
  Food Pyramid and, 54–55
  kickoff, 49–51
  personalizing your, 51–52
  point system, 54
  on the road, 60
  shopping and cooking for, 58–60

educational program
   American Diabetes Association and, 139
   books/booklets for, 140
   books for home library, 143–144
   hospital or community center sources, 139–140
   on Internet, 142
   magazines and newsletters for, 143
   phone book for, 140
   responsibility for self, 136
   support groups, 136–137
emotions
   attitude adjustment, 39–41
   blood glucose levels and, 36
   physical activity and, 39
   stress and, 36–41
Ergoset, 79
estrogen
   symptoms of lack of, 111–112
exchange system, 52
   advantages of, 52
   Healthy Food Choices program, 52
exercise
   aerobic, 70
   age and, 69–70
   anaerobic, 70
   benefits of, 63
   blood glucose levels and, 30–31
   blood glucose monitoring and, 101
   calories burned by, 73
   as coping strategy for stress, 39
   excuses not to, 64
   eye problems and, 68–69
   flexibility exercises, 70
   formal exercise program, 65–66, 71–72
   goals for, 65
   heart and kidney problems, 69

historical perspective for diabetes management, 21

hypoglycemia, 30–31

intensive, 71–72

listening to body, 68

moderately intense workout, 21

monitoring blood glucose levels and, 67

neuropathy and, 68

with partner, 66

pet and, 66–67

physical activity options for, 72–73

regular exercise options, 70–71

several short periods daily, 21, 64, 138

tracking progress in diary, 67

variety of, 64

eye problems. *See also* retinopathy

exercise and, 68–69

F

fasting

in kickoff eating plan, 50

fat

body's need for, 47

in diet, 90

figure percentage of calories from fat, 57

food choices and, 47

in kickoff eating plan, 50–51

fiber

carbohydrate counting and, 53

food choices, 48

flexibility exercise, 70

food choices

alcohol, 48–49

best for diabetes, 139

carbohydrates and, 47–48

childhood patterns and, 44

cookbooks and, 61

eating out, 60

fiber, 48

figure percentage of calories from fat, 57

healthy portions and, 49

historical perspective for treatment, 20–21

importance of, 43

kickoff eating plan, 50

portion size, 57

protein, 46–47

reading food labels and, 57–58

on the road, 60

sodium, 48

speed to convert to blood glucose and, 43

sugar and, 47–48

sweeteners and, 47–48

total fat and, 47

for weight loss, 46

food labels

reading, 57–58

Food Pyramid

eating plan and, 54–55

Forecast, 143

fructosamine test, 103

fructose, 48

G

gestational diabetes, 23, 26, 151

Glimepiride, 76, 80

Glipizide, 76, 81

glucagon, 124

uses of, 145

Glucophage, 77, 81

glucose

defined, 145

insulin and normal working of, 29

purpose of, 145

Glucotrol, 76, 81

Glyburide, 76, 81

glycemic index system, 56

glycosylated hemoglobin, 103

   defined, 145

   normal reading of, 146

   purpose of, 145–146

Glynase, 76, 81

Glyset, 78, 81

H

Healthy Food Choices program, 52

heart disease

   as complication of diabetes, 127–129

   exercise and, 69

hemoglobin A1c, 145–146

high blood glucose, 32–33, 125–126. *See also* hyperglycemia

   damage from, 32–33

   signs and symptoms of, 126

   symptoms of, 32

high carbohydrate, high fiber (HCF) system, 56

HOE, 82

hyperglycemia, 24, 125–126. *See also* high blood glucose

   defined, 146

   range of, 146

   signs and symptoms of, 126

   symptoms of, 146–147

hypertension

   as complication of diabetes, 127–129

   medication for, 87–90

hypertrophy

   defined, 147

hypoglycemia, 19, 123–125. *See also* low blood glucose

   defined, 147

   emergency treatment for, 124

   exercise and, 30–31

range of, 147

signs and symptoms of, 124–125

symptoms of, 147

treatment for, 124, 148

I

illnesses

blood glucose levels and, 31

imaging, 37

impaired glucose tolerance, 23, 151

impotence, 33

impotency, 116–119

nerve damage and, 117–118

treatment fro, 118–119

information program

American Diabetes Association and, 139

books/booklets for, 140

books for home library, 143–144

hospital or community center sources, 139–140

on Internet, 142

magazines and newsletters for, 143

phone book for, 140

responsibility for self, 136

support groups, 136–137

insulin, 82–86

action of available, 83

assistive devices for, 85–86

automatic injector, 85

balancing eating and exercise with, 82–83

blood glucose levels response to, 31

defined, 148

disposing of needles, 84

function of, 82

inhaled, 79, 82

injecting, 84

insulin pen, 85

insulin pump, 85

    normal working of, 29

    pre-meal blood glucose information, 86

    proper storage of, 86

    rotating injection sites, 84

    spray injector, 85

    strength of, 84

    syringe sizes for, 84

    types of, 138, 148

insulin-dependent diabetes mellitus, 23, 26

    defined, 148–149

insulin reaction, 123–125

    emergency treatment for, 124

    signs and symptoms of, 124–125

    treatment for, 124

insulin resistance, 29, 82

insulin sensitivity enhancers, 78–79

International Diabetes Center

    addresses and phone numbers for, 141

Internet

    diabetes information on, 142

IUD (Intrauterine Device), 115

J

Joslin Diabetes Center

    addresses and phone numbers for, 141

journal

    advantages of, 131

    disadvantages of, 132

    for exercise, 67

    list of basic information to record in, 132–133

Juvenile Diabetes Foundation

    addresses and phone numbers for, 141

juvenile-onset diabetes, 23

K

ketosis/ketoacidosis, 24, 125, 147
  defined, 149
  untreated, 147
  urine test for, 102–103
kickoff eating plan, 49–51
  carbohydrates in, 50
  fats in, 50–51
  three-day fast, 50
kidney problems. *See also* nephropathy
    as complication of diabetes, 129–130
  exercise and, 69

L

lactic acidosis, 77
lipoatrophy
  defined, 149
long-term complications, 126–130
low blood glucose, 31–32, 123–125. *See also* hypoglycemia
  emergency treatment for, 124
  signs and symptoms of, 124–125
  symptoms of, 31
  treatment for, 124

M

magazines on diabetes, 143
medication
  arthritis and pain, 91–92
  cholesterol and triglyceride, 90–91
  cough and cold, 92
  for hypertension, 87–90
  insulin, 82–86
  oral hypoglycemic agents, 75–82
  other medication, 87
meditation, 37
meglitinides, 79

men's issues
  impotency, 116–119
  sexuality, 116–119
metformin, 77, 81
Micronase, 76, 81
miglitol, 78, 81
monitoring health. *See* blood glucose monitoring

N

National Diabetes Information Clearinghouse
  addresses and phone numbers for, 141
nephropathy
  as complication of diabetes, 129–130
  defined, 149–150
neuropathy, 32, 97
  autonomic, 130, 150
  as complication of diabetes, 130
  defined, 150
  exercise and, 68
  impotency and, 117–118
  peripheral, 130, 150
newsletters on diabetes, 143
noninsulin-dependent diabetes mellitus, 23, 150–152
  treatment for, 151
nonsteroid anti-inflammatory drug, 91–92
Norplant, 114

O

oral hypoglycemic agents, 25, 75–82
  alpha-glucosidase inhibitors, 78
  biguanides, 77
  blood glucose levels, 31
  defined, 152
  historical background of, 75–76
  meglitinides, 79
  names of specific agents, dosages and duration, 80–81

sulfonylureas, 76–77
thiazolidinediones, 78–79
for Type 1 diabetes, 24
Orinase, 76, 80
osteoporosis, 112–113

P

pain medication, 91–92
peripheral neuropathy, 150
Pill, 114
point system eating plan, 54
portion control, 49, 57
Prandin, 79, 81
Precose, 78, 81
pregnancy, 113
progesterone
    symptoms of lack of, 111–112
proliferative retinopathy, 129, 153
protein
    food choices and, 46–47

R

renal threshold
    defined, 152
    range for, 152
repaglinide, 79, 81
retinopathy, 33, 97
    background, 129, 153
    cause of, 152
    defined, 152–153
    proliferative, 129, 153
Rezulin, 78–79, 81
rhythm method of birth control, 115
rosiglitazone maleate, 79

S

sexuality, 109–119
  birth control options, 114–116
  blood glucose levels and, 110
  female issues of, 110–113
  impotency, 116–119
  menopause and aging, 111–112
  men's issues, 116–119
  pregnancy, 113
  vaginal infections, 110
short-term complications, 123–126
smoking, 113
  aging and, 111
sodium
  decreasing amount, 59–60
  food choices and, 48
sponge, birth control, 115
stress
  acupuncture, 39
  attitude adjustment, 39–41
  biofeedback, 38
  blood glucose levels and, 31, 36, 101
  coping strategies for, 37–41
  imaging, 37
  learning about, 37
  meditation, 37
  physical activity and, 39
  tips for handling, 36
strokes
  as complication of diabetes, 127–129
sugar
  as cause of diabetes, 27
  decreasing amount, 59
  eating as part of meal, 137–138
  food choices and, 47–48
sulfonylureas, 76–77

sweeteners

food choices and, 47–48

sweets

eating as part of meal, 137–138

T

Targretin, 79

thiazolidinediones, 78–79

tight blood glucose control programs

benefits of, 12–13, 97–98, 121–122, 123

starting one, 122–123

Tolazamide, 76, 80

Tolbutamide, 76, 80

Tolinase, 76, 80

total available glucose (TAG) system, 56

triglyceride medication, 90–91

troglitazone, 78–79, 81

tubal ligation, 115–116

Type 1 diabetes, 23

cause of, 24, 149

characteristics of, 23–24

complications of, 24

defined, 148–149

insulin and, 148

management plan for, 24

oral hypoglycemic agents, 24

Type 2 diabetes

body weight and, 25

characteristics of, 24–25

complications of, 26

defined, 150

diabetes management program, 25–26

genetic tendency for, 25

insulin and, 148

prevalence of, 150

treatment for, 151

U

urine ketone test, 102–103
urine sugar test, 102

V

vaginal infections, 110
vasectomy, 115
Viagra, 119
vision problems. *See* retinopathy

W

weight
  checking weekly, 133
  Type 2 diabetes and, 25
weight control
  childhood patterns and, 44
weight loss
  benefit of, 27
  better food choices for, 46
  blood glucose monitoring and, 101–102
  over reasonable period of time, 45, 46
withdrawal method of birth control, 115
women's issues
  menopause and aging, 111–112
  osteoporosis, 112–113
  pregnancy, 113
  vaginal infections, 110

Y

yohimbine, 119
yo-yo dieting syndrome, 45